But Serioulsy,

WHERE DID THE TIME GO?

A TEENAGE JOURNEY OF TRIUMPH OVER ACUTE LYMPHOBLASTIC LYMPHOMA

JETHRO R. PIERRE

In partnership with the following Consulting Editors: Hermeline Blanc & Paigelawson216@Fiverr.com.

ISBN-13: 978-0-9894680-8-4 (paperback)

Published by:
Divine Works Publishing, LLC.
Royal Palm Beach, Florida USA

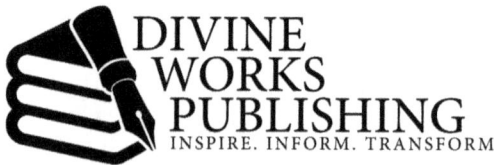

DIVINE
WORKS
PUBLISHING
INSPIRE. INFORM. TRANSFORM

www.DivineWorksPublishing.com
561-990-BOOK (2665)

Acknowledgments

Nephtalie Pierre, thank you for always guiding and supporting me with everything I've pursued in life. You have always given me the most loving, blunt, crucial advice on everything in life, especially for this book. You always have kept me in check on being credible and spiritual as a young adult.

Carmie Pierre, thank you for protecting me and taking care of me your whole life. To the point where you literally gave me a piece of your physical body. I think at this point I've driven you crazy and you are done with me.

Dad, I don't know how you did it. You sacrificed nearly everything to come here from Haiti and create this wonderful family. Only to watch it all fall apart. Then to bring it back together again even better than before. It should have been you writing this book instead of me! You've always put others ahead of you, no matter the consequences. You've done everything and beyond for our family. I love you dad.

I would like to thank Belinda John and the entire Divine Works Publishing team for helping me with this book and see it come to a finished work.

I would like thank POST for always going the extra mile for my family and I.

Thank you to all of my family and friends who supported me and assisted me throughout this project. You all have a special place in my heart: Ian Derosa, Mikey Marrone, Matthew George, Hermline Blanc, Sadrack Mentor, Anthony Munoz, Jephte Blanc, Yvelor Sully, Pastor Moise, Julie Lanosa, Albert Torres, Gabriel Vazquez, Elizabeth Espinosa, Elizabeth Cardona, Maddison Mackenzie, Lauren Tavares, Victoria Vazquez, Patrick Kolta, Alex Vazquez, Mardoshee Mercius, Kitty, My dogs Squanto and Lickie for lifting my spirits, and everyone else who loved and supported me throughout this journey, there are too many names to mention them all.

Dedication

Marie Pierre

I can't seem to get out of your arms... I've been in them since January 23, 1997, since breastfeeding, since you were studying your nursing book with me in your lap while I ripped out pages from your books, since dropping me off at daycare and me not wanting to leave, since crying after that bookshelf fell on me, since getting my first soccer medal in Wellington, since falling asleep on you in church almost every Sunday, since crying from getting bullied by my sisters, since playing travel soccer, since my first day of high school, since my first failing grade, since my first date, since graduation, since my first job, since my diagnosis of cancer. I dedicate this book to you because I know it will always be in your arms; like I will continue to be.

Contents

Prologue by Nephtalie Pierre
Jethro's oldest sister

On January 23, 1997, my parents were blessed with a baby boy. He was wrapped in love, peace, joy and carried on the backs of my parents' (Roosevelt and Marie Pierre) prayers. We welcome him to the world with a room full of aunts, uncles, cousins, doctors, and nurses; my father, my younger sister, Carmie, and myself. We named him Jethro Roosevelt Pierre, hoping he would positively impact the world and honor our family.

He grew up to be a curious and rambunctious boy who knew exactly what he wanted and refused to take no for an answer. As he grew, he turned to Carmie and me, his older sisters, for guidance on expressing himself. We taught him what we could, keeping a mental note of his odd behaviors. What kid thinks about effective communication at such a young age? As he grew, his circle of friends also grew. In a short time, he mastered the art of communication and was effective at reaching people. People loved him.

There were a few unforgettable moments. For example, my brother told me that he would like to get baptized. I thought he was weird. In retrospect, he was not weird at all. Instead, he developed a thirst for something more. A few months later, my brother and I went to church. I had no idea God was preparing me for this day. I thought we were late for service. But little did we know, we both had an appointment to reconnect with God. I was proud of my brother that day. Since then, I have watched my brother grow in faith.

Seemingly insignificant but memorable moments like when Jethro picked on me about my television addiction engraved in my heart. He did not like my Lifetime movie Saturdays, Oxygen's Snapped Sundays, and in between how

I binge-watched Golden Girls, my favorite T.V. shows.

I first watched the Golden Girls episode "Ebbtide's Revenge," where Sophia's son, Dorothy's younger brother, Phil, dies. Dorothy delivered a loving and memorable eulogy in which she humbly expressed:

> "It seems like I'm always mad at my brother Phil. I was angry the day my parents brought him back from the hospital. I thought he'd take their love away from me, and instead, their love expanded, and we felt more like a family. I was mad at him when I was ten, and he was four, and we moved to a new neighborhood. I was mad because he always made new friends more easily than I did. And I'm mad today because I never wanted to give the eulogy at my kid brother's funeral. I'm mad because he died. He didn't have the wisdom to know that family members shouldn't allow themselves to grow apart. Because when this day comes, they can no longer tell each other how they care. If he'd had that wisdom, he could have shared it with me, and I would have known the hundreds of memories I have of just the two of us."

Rewind the clock to when I first watched that episode at 14. I looked at my 5-year older brother Jethro as tears clouded my vision; I prayed never to be put in Dorothy's position. I thought, "No. Not me... I couldn't let him go." I must have watched this episode a dozen times after that.

Like Dorothy, it seemed as if I was always mad at my brother. I was angry that he would take away all my parent's love from me, that he made friends easier than me, and that I had to give his eulogy at the fruitful age of 21. My brother was wise enough to understand, experience, and cherish love with his friends and family.

Today, I carry in my heart stories from people who were once strangers to my brother's kindness, love, and genuine nature. Those stories provide comfort and assurance that my brother positively impacted his world. I feel privileged to observe the love poem God wrote to my brother with tightly woven blessings disguised as random coincidences throughout his life. I could hear God say, "Oh how I love thee, Jethro, let me count the ways." He commands day and time to express much love to you, Jethro!

In the end, we had so many wishes for Jethro. Words we wanted to say, places we wanted to go, and moments we wanted to share. So, the enclosed journal entries are dedicated to you, my brother Jethro Pierre. To finish the work you started, to our family, to the love we share, to the battle we face, to the journey we take, and to the lessons we learned.

This journal is an example of his love. My brother Jethro smiles light the room with every opportunity to share his story. He hoped that his life would affect someone and take him places. I know he would have been proud of his work and to know that his fight was not in vain. He has won because he is no longer suffering; his words, which you are about to read, are now being shared. Jethro's story of love, fearlessness, and fight, written in his words, will impact your own story. I say Glory to the highest and pray that God demonstrates this same love to you with every word and turning pages. What a privilege to have had a front-row seat into his life's experiences and the love that he shares.

Disclaimer

This journal depicts the life and experiences of the author, Jethro R. Pierre. Some names have been changed to honor and respect his friends and family's privacy. Although some storylines have been altered to conceal the identity of the characters, major themes and events are based on real-life events journaled by the author, Jethro R. Pierre.

Chapter One

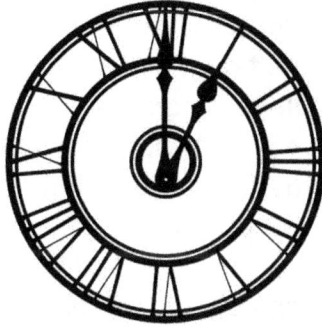

THE INCIDENT
November 2015

My life is nothing short of a mistake. I lived in a modest family home in West Palm Beach, FL, with my parents and siblings for the first three years. Later, we moved to the Village of Wellington, where I played soccer until I was 18, both as a travel and high school soccer player. My stellar sportsmanship led me to play for the state of Florida Olympic Development Program. But if you ask my family, they remember my early days on the soccer field. They lovingly teased me because of my round eyeglasses. Imagine a skinny little "Steve Urkle" running around the soccer field with a ball. My family joked that I initially lacked the toughness to play sports because I refused to play rough. But that did not last. I became an avid player on my team. Soccer runs in my blood since I am of Haitian descent and my father's son.

My father, Roosevelt Pierre, was an avid soccer player in his home country of Haiti. He gave up his dream of playing for the Haitian National Football (Soccer) Team to pursue the American dream. My mother, Marie Odette Mercius, the first out of her family to immigrate to the U.S. As with most immigrant families, my parents worked long hours, so my two older sisters, Nephtalie and Carmie, helped my parents take care of me. My life revolved around soccer, school, church, and family during those early years. By the time I got to high school, I was a star player and a leading scorer.

> God kept our family together through a lot. He kept us together even through the hardest of times.

My senior year of high school was my year of freedom. It was the best! By this time, my sisters and three of my older cousins, who lived with us for a time, left for college to follow their dreams and aspirations. It was just me, mom, dad, and the dogs (Lickie and Squanto).

In high school, classes were easy. I increased my GPA my senior year. I got my first car (Scion TC 2011) and had some great friends—the chorus squad—as many of us were in choir together. I had my first girlfriend. Although I went to my senior prom alone, I had fun, and it was a night to remember.

But all that changed after high school; I fell into a slight depression because my dream of playing college soccer did not come true as no college offered me a viable scholarship. I played it safe with my parents' guidance and attended Palm Beach State. I got two jobs and adjusted to college life.

Little did I know, I was not ready for reality. One night, while writing an essay for my English class, I took a quick break to get a drink and use the bathroom. While looking in the mirror, I noticed a swollen Cheetos-shaped, hard lump under my right ear at the side of my jawline. I ran upstairs, woke my mom, and showed her the bump. She looked at it and said, "You should go to the pediatric office tomorrow." So, the next day, I went to the doctor, and he suspected that I had infectious mononucleosis, commonly known as mono or the kissing disease. He shared that the symptoms of mono do not appear until 4 to 6 weeks. In the meantime, he advised that I should not work or go to the gym. He said the lump should disappear on its own.

But it did not. Instead, another one grew on the other side of my head. So, my mom and I went back to the doctor. The doctor still did not think it was anything to be concerned about, but he referred us to an Ear, Nose, and Throat doctor (ENT) specialist. At the ENT clinic, the doctor examined me and observed that I was getting these lumps in different places—under my chin, neck, elbow, and pelvis. He did a needle aspiration from the lump behind my ear. I learned that these lumps are called lymph nodes and are all over our bodies. Sometimes when one is sick, they rise to help fight colds and infections, then usually go down once the person is feeling better. But mine never went down. The lymph nodes sample from the needle aspiration showed Lymphoma—a potentially cancerous infection.

The ENT doctor ordered a lymph node biopsy on the side of my neck because it was the smallest lump. Also, it causes the least complications. The surgery was set to be done on the following Saturday. Over that week, I did three blood tests, which I was getting tired of. I told my mom I hate needles. She said if this were cancer, I would have to get used to it. She told me to speak to my friend Luis, who survived cancer, about how hard it could be and about how many blood tests he went through.

I got the point. Saturday morning soon arrived. On the drive there, my mom explained everything that would happen. She urged me not to be scared and reassured me that everything would be alright. I told her I was fine even though I was utterly terrified inside.

We got there, checked in, and went to the pre-operation room. The nurses told me to change into my gown, asked me if I ate, placed the heart monitor on my chest, and then stuck an IV in my hand. It didn't hurt as much as my mom said it would. My mom held my hand as we waited for the anesthesia specialist and the ENT doctor to arrive. The nurse was concerned because my heart levels were off and said I needed to relax and get comfortable. I was scared out of my mind. Like a mama's boy, I asked my mom to sing one of those Haitian hymns she sang to me as a kid. It was a corny moment, but it helped me relax.

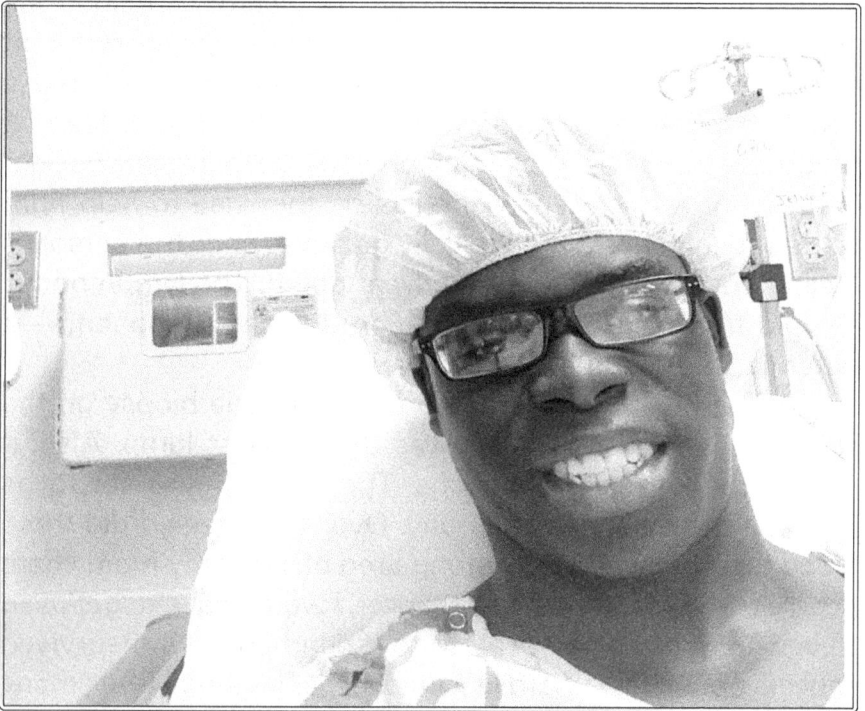

The anesthesia kicked in and knocked me out. The procedure went fine.

We went through the weekend hoping that the results would come back negative. But when Monday came, the results shocked us to the core. My mother's instinct was right. She received a phone call from the ENT Doctor confirming my diagnosis. The result was cancerous. My mom didn't want to tell me, so I pried it out of her. I started to tear up, but I forced myself to stop. I promised myself to cry no matter how hard things get. I was diagnosed with a rare form of aggressive Non-Hodgkin T-lymphoblastic lymphoma.

Suddenly, my mom was forced to seek out the best place to receive treatments. My priorities changed overnight. I had to tell my family and friends I had cancer. I'm a very friendly person, which I get from my father. In my young life, I had a lot of close friends, whether it was at the mall, the gym, at church; I was very close with my teachers at school, my co-workers, and even closer with my family. The people I care about need to know, but how do I tell them? I did not want things to change. I did not want them to think I could be dying and worry about me. I did not want them to treat me differently. They would begin to go soft on me. Start seeing me as a sick, dying person. I did not want that! I did not want to accept that lifestyle. I wished there was a way to tell them I had cancer while keeping everything the same.

By Thursday of that week, I was so stressed. I did not care about anything. All I wanted to do was work out since I had not gone to the gym for about three weeks. Two of my closest friends came with me. I felt safe enough to run on the treadmill. I ran at high speeds for about 40 minutes, blasting music and trying to clear my mind. I was running so fast; one would have thought I was trying to run this cancer out of me.

Afterward, while at Chick-Fil-A, I told them both. They were shocked and sad for me. At first, one of my friends did

> Lymphoma is the most common blood cancer with two main forms of lymphoma: Hodgkin lymphoma and non-Hodgkin lymphoma (NHL). Lymphoma occurs when cells of the immune system called lymphocytes, a type of white blood cell, grow and multiply uncontrollably.
> –The Lymphoma Research Foundation

5

not believe it; I emphasized.

The next day, I went to see an Oncology doctor. As we waited in the lobby, my mind went wild as I saw many people with cancer looking old and frail. I thought to myself, would that be me soon? Do any of these people know that I am the one that is sick and not my mom? How much time is on my clock? I am sure there is a lot more these older people have accomplished. If they die, they can say they lived a great long life. I just got out of high school. Will I get to experience college life, play collegiate soccer, graduate college, learn new languages, be successful, be in a steady relationship, buy a house, get married, see the world, have kids, or even help my parents retire? I also thought that although things were bad right now, it did not mean I couldn't do anything about it.

Finally, the nurse brought me back to reality as she called us to see the doctor. I felt a slight relief but still pondered all those questions, and the future awaited me. The nurse drew my blood as usual. I got used to it. A good trick is not to look. The doctor came in and confirmed the results of my neck lymph node biopsy. He then told us he could treat me locally in a nearby hospital. But then he said, if you want the best treatment and the best doctors in America, you should go to Dana-Farber Cancer Institute in Boston. They can completely wipe out your cancer, and they always get great results." So, my mom said she would drop everything: her new job, school as she was working toward her B.A. in nursing, and her church activities to fly me out to Boston the next day. The receptionist at the clinic gave us instructions on what to do once we arrived there.

After the appointment, I dropped my mom off at work. I could not think during the ride home; my head was everywhere. I did not know what to do.

I was mad that this was all happening to me. I was heated. I felt like I needed a way to control what was happening and find a way to express my feelings. So, I decided to start a journal. I went to Walmart got a journal, pens, and sharpies. Again, I thought because things are bad right now does not mean I could not do anything about it. Journaling was the only way I felt in control of what was happening to me.

I left for Boston the next day, and most of my close family and friends didn't even know I had cancer. I texted my childhood friends to meet up at my best friend Jordan's house. They played 2K (an American video game) when I got there. I realized how much I would miss them. I told them to pause the game because I could not stay long and quickly explained the situation. I was perplexed and wanted to cry but be strong for my friends.

> Just because things are bad right now doesn't mean I can't do anything about it.

While packing, I called everyone on my contact list. I gave them the news, and almost all of them did not believe me at first. Some cried; some did not. One of my friends prayed with me on the phone. He told me that this sickness does not have a hold on me. His prayer stayed with me for a while. Through each call, I stayed strong and positive. I told everyone that I would be okay and that I did not know how long I'd be gone.

I jumped in my car to go to the mall to pick up my sister Carmie. While driving to the mall, I called Mr. Houchins, my high school chorus teacher, and it was the first time I cried. I could not breathe or talk straight. I was very emotional speaking to the man who helped me discover my musical gift and my extrovert personality. He helped make all four years of high school enjoyable. He changed my life.

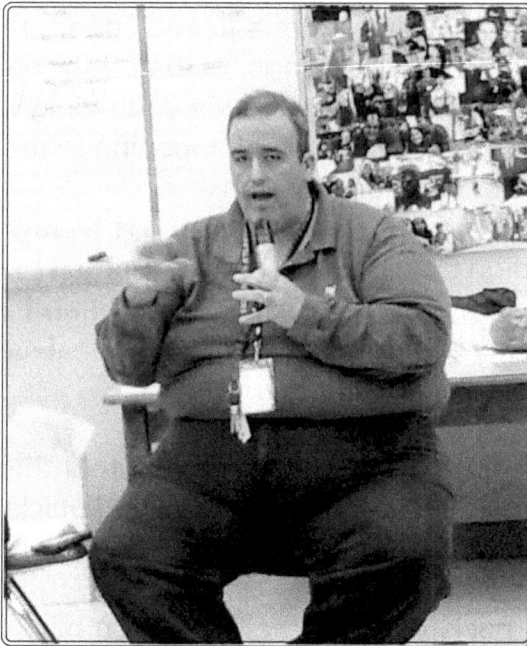

Mr. Houchins
Director of Choral Activities at Palm Beach Central High
Performing Arts Chair at School District of Palm Beach

After picking up my sister, it was a quiet drive home. Everything was happening so quickly. We were both scared. What is there to say? I got home. My aunts and cousins were there. I said hi to everyone, gave them hugs and kisses, and told them that I'd be back. Besides, my mom would share more of the details. I went outside and finished my calls.

I got a call from my friend Luis, who was diagnosed with Lymphoma years earlier, was in complete remission and cure. I told him what was happening, and he said we needed to see each other as soon as possible. I met him at the Walmart parking lot. He did not seem as worried as I thought he would be. He shared how he cried when he first heard I had cancer. He also told me that he was not concerned about me because he knew my great personality and belief in God would help me through it. He reached in his pocket, pulled out a necklace pendant of Jesus on the cross, and handed it to me. He told me it would take a long time for him to say everything he wanted me to know. But he shared that it is more mental than physical throughout this process and to use the cross to help me. He reiterated that I would be okay, and he loved me. I was confused but deeply touched and grateful.

My sisters helped me find two expensive airplane tickets for an early morning flight. Money was the least of our concerns. It is funny how our priority shifted regarding life and death situations.

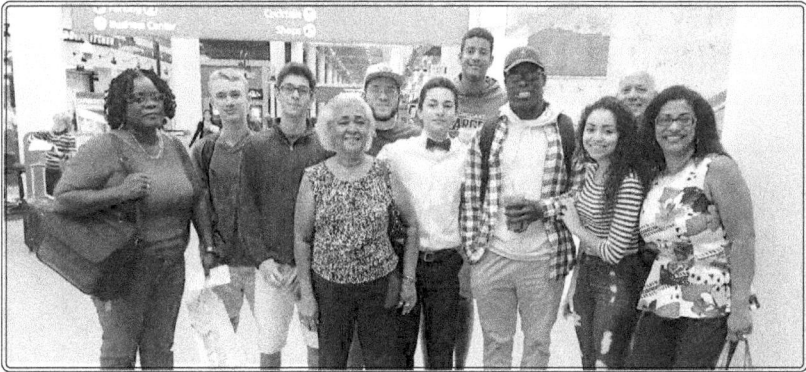

The following day, at the Palm Beach International Airport, a few friends and their parents gathered to say goodbye before mom, and I left for Boston. As we reached security clearance, I said bye to everyone one by one. I hugged my dad, feeling like I failed in life. My main goal was to succeed in soccer for him. He sacrificed so much for our family. Leaving a professional soccer career, he moved here from Haiti to start a new life, one with more promise. I held back my tears as I hugged him. I wanted to cry my eyes out, but I had to stay strong again. I waved goodbye as I walked through the rails behind my mom and handed the security agent my ticket. I heard someone scream, "Jethro, wait!". I turned back, and two of my friends were with their mom. I hugged them as they cried, like everyone before them. Iyana handed me a small devotional booklet which kept me sane throughout the entire journey in Boston. I said one last goodbye to everyone, gave the security personnel my ticket, and stopped for a second look. I held on to the railing and breathed so hard. My mom asked if I was okay. I told her, "You don't know the pain I'm feeling right now." My heart was wrecked, having to leave my life behind with no idea of what awaited me.

Chapter Two

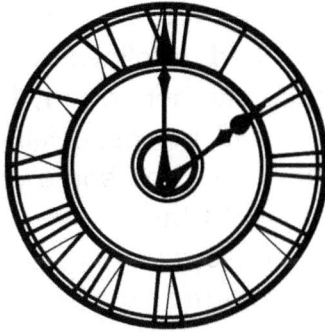

THE NEWS
December 2015 ~ Days 1-14

We reached Boston safely and took the taxi to Dana-Farber Cancer Institute, where they ran several tests. Finally, we met the doctors who schooled my mom and me about my disease. The doctor said Lymphoma is curable and that my chances of survival are high. Then, they dropped the bomb on us, "Your chances of having kids decreased significantly with chemotherapy," followed by the words that pierced my heart, "you'll have to bank sperm before you start chemo." I left the room for a few minutes to pull myself together. I always wanted a little "Monty" or "Anne." After much contemplation, I decided to adopt if I could not have any children.

Although I was 18, the doctors thought it was best to treat me as a child because survival rates are higher in children. They transferred me across the street to Boston Children's Hospital Hematology and Oncology. They took my vitals and drew my blood again. Once we were assigned to a room, the nurse placed a more extensive IV in my left forearm, which hurt. I fell asleep on the small bed while my mom slept on an uncomfortable chair, waiting for them to prepare a bigger room.

After an hour or so, the nurse told us our room was ready. We were exhausted. We rushed to get our bags together. I climbed out of bed to follow, but the nurse stopped me and said they'd take me there on my bed. As they transported me, I saw many patients, especially teenagers around my age. They looked terrible, and some were screaming like their lives were ending right there. I was terrified the rest of the way up, so I closed my eyes and prayed.

We made it to the room on the fifth floor without speaking. My mom thought I was sleeping. The next day, we were moved up to the sixth floor. To keep me hydrated, the nurse connected my IV to fluids. The room we were in was better than I expected. The bathroom was clean. The food was decent there. My mom slept on the windowsill bed, which I hated because I did not want her to be uncomfortable. But she said it was fine.

At first, I didn't want to accept what was happening. I didn't want to research my disease. I didn't want to speak to survivors. I kept thinking of all the things I would be missing out on: going to the movies, swimming pools, and parties because I was stuck in the hospital. Life changes for people with cancer.

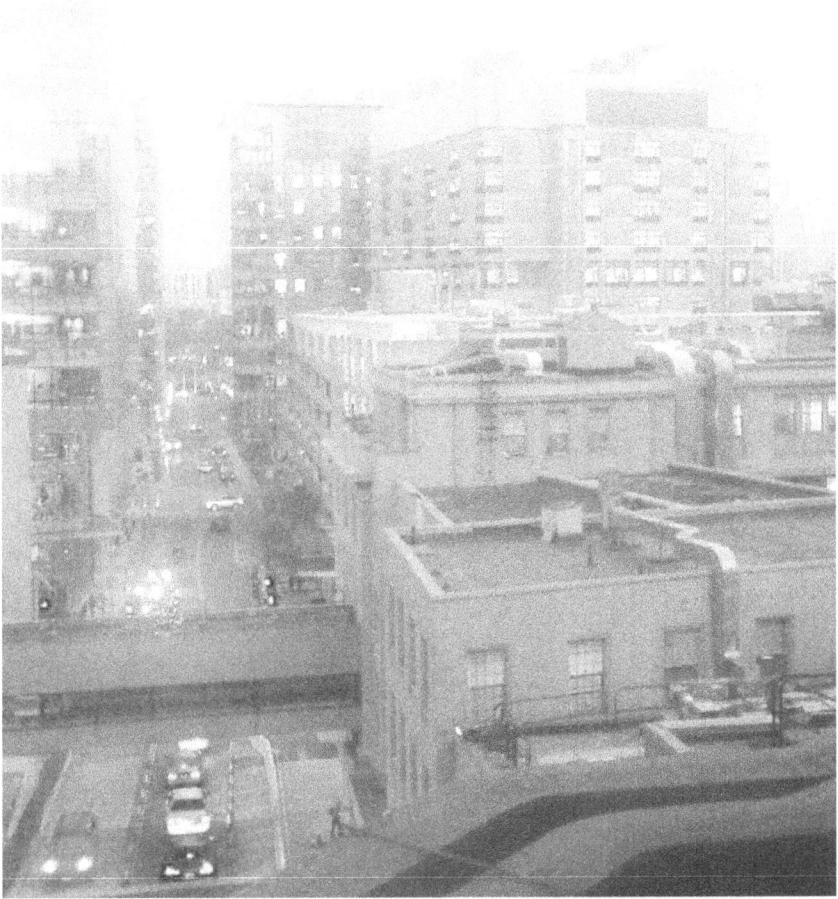

My Window View from Boston Hospital.
Boston Longwood Blackfan Street

As I got ready for bed, I decided to use my own experience in a way that could be helpful to others, especially the many scared teenagers. Every night, I wrote in my journal and read pages from the devotional that my friend Iyana gave me and touched the pendant Luis gifted me.

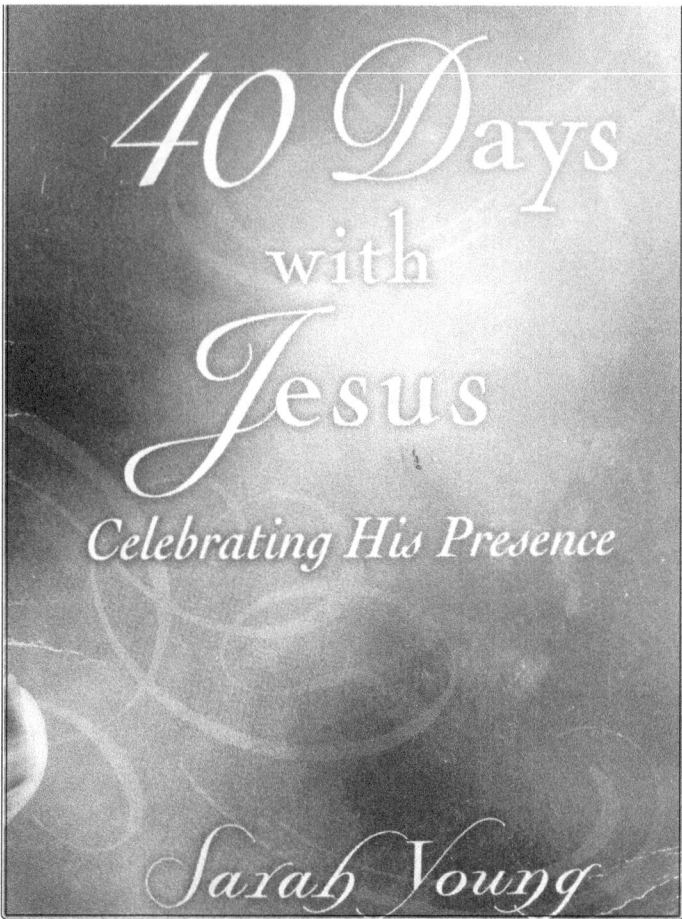

*No matter how good or bad my day is,
I will do this because my story can help another life.*

I cannot explain how I felt or whether I feared the coming days at Boston Children's Hospital. One thing I knew for sure was that God was on my side and was not putting me through in vain. I learned that God never wants to hurt us or put us through any pain. All the negativity and pain Jesus Christ took on the cross and conquered for us was not in vain.

So, when an IV goes into my body or when I go through

painful operations, I think of Jesus Christ. He has already endured all my pain and sins.

Every day leading up to my chemo was important. It determined how strong I would be during it. I needed to keep a positive mindset because I knew I would not feel like myself. Before I left Florida, my cousin Yvelor shared his belief in the law of attraction; he said if I do not feel sick, I am not sick. If I do not think I am sick, I'm not sick. This means that whatever thoughts I have will manifest in real life. If I believe I will come across a good fortune, I will come across a good fortune. If I think bad things will happen to my health, bad things will happen. I kept those words close to my heart.

During the first couple of days in Boston, I questioned my feelings about everything. There were days when I was terrified. There were days I was super hyper. At times, I could not understand how I felt just fine but was sick. To cure me, the proper treatment would make me sicker. How is flushing my body with medicine that made me sicker the most logical way to heal me? I could not understand.

The happiest and most hopeful I felt was when Joy, one of my mom's closest friends who happened to be a nurse and live in Boston, visited us. She encouraged me and told me that everything happens for a reason and that Boston's Children's Hospital is the best hospital to be at when you're sick. She joked, "Jethro, you are in heaven."

One of the most challenging questions and mysteries is how I ended up with cancer. My mom and my family struggled most with this question as well. She looked everywhere for answers. She thought it could have been the artificial turf grass I played soccer on, pesticides, or radiation exposure. Unfortunately, we will never figure out what exactly caused me to have Non-Hodgkin's Lymphoblastic lymphoma.

It was hard for me to believe that I, an avid 18-year-old soccer player with a long life ahead of me, ended up with cancer. My thoughts became so ridiculous and irrational that I started to blame myself for my diagnosis. So, you mean when I got in trouble in public school at eight for stealing candy and being transferred to private school led to this? Do you mean playing the Trombone in sixth grade and deciding to stop because I feel it made my lips too big led to this? Is getting teased because of my race led to this? Is not having a girlfriend until senior year and finding out she wasn't the one led to this? Is not having a date for senior prom led to this? Is wasting 15 years as a soccer player and not being selected by a college to play soccer led to this? Is being born on 01/23/97? I concluded that everything wrong that ever happened up to this point led to my cancer diagnosis. When you have no answer for something unexplainable, you try to find someone or something to blame. And if there are no rational answers, we tend to point the finger internally.

The fact is I am a freshman in college who is actively working out, making music, having a decent paying job, and a long life ahead of him. I did not want to believe this was happening to me. I did not have time for this! My only option was to take each step, one at a time. Think positive and keep my head up. After much deliberation, I thought God planned for this, God will get me through this, and God has a reward for me when I win this battle. There is something bigger than I can imagine. And trust me, my imagination runs wild. God put every great man in the bible through a test. I believe this is mine.

> God planned for this; God will get me through this. God has a reward for me when I win this battle.

I expected painful IVs, surgery, and terrible medications. I was not feeling too good either. Every four hours, a nurse came in and checked my vitals. I attempted to write a song called "Check my vitals" using that analogy; some people did not care to check up on me until they found out I was sick. I stopped because it wasn't helping me stay positive.

I also blamed myself because my mom dropped everything to be with me. I love her so much. I do not know what

I'd do without her. However, I haven't shown it enough. Many times, I did not prioritize her feelings and understand her intentions. For example, I got frustrated because she went over my long to-do list with me. She could read it on my face. I was not motivated. She asked if she was annoying me, and I rudely answered, "No!" I thought, "I am not even on meds, and we are already having problems." I love my mom so much and didn't want to change while I was on meds and start snapping at her. She means so much to me.

My good friend, Niafa, was also on my mind. She is the type of person to bring you up whenever you are down. That day, she tried to encourage me. She said that there is no way all my friends will let those medications get the best of me. But I thought, "Well, how can you help me? If I do not want to talk, I can turn off my phone. You're all so far from me."

Mom advised me to open the little package Iyana gave to me at the airport. The box was filled with great scripture about fighting cancer with the power of God. That is when I realized that I will always have God help me through my troubles wherever I go. My mom was by my side singing hymns from her "Chants D'esperance" (Haitian hymn book), and my aunts were texting weeks' worth of bible verses to me.

On the fourth day of my treatment, one of the first lymph nodes in my neck sored all day. The next day, I got a Peripherally Inserted Central Catheter (PICC) line procedure done in my arm so they could start my chemotherapy. I mostly slept through it.

> *That's when I realized wherever I go, I will always have God helping me through my troubles.*

I had a lumbar puncture done. I banked sperm and had a Positron Emission Tomography (PET) pet scan. Banking sperm was the weirdest and most uncomfortable thing I've ever done in my entire life. The room was sketchy and dimmed. Some magazines were foreign to me. The PET scan, however, was not too bad.

The weirdest part was the liquid they put through my IV to see in my body. The liquid made inside of my body feel warm. I received steroids every day as the primary drug. I walked around and felt fine after the procedures, but the treatments had me feeling down again. What cheered me up was the portable piano delivered to my room. I requested it because I wanted to learn to play while stuck in the hospital. I wrote a song.

After preparing, I returned to my room and saw my mom crying. I comforted her. It is going to be hard for both of us.

My cousin Hermeline visited me from New Jersey for Thanksgiving after three years of not seeing each other. Since she could not go back to Florida, she decided to make the five-hour drive to Boston to spend the holiday with my mom and me. The hospital had a huge Thanksgiving lunch for everyone! We did a lot of walking. Boston Children's Hospital is so big that it has its own radio station (Seacrest Studios). I would love to be there live on-air and play my music. We relaxed, played cards, and watched a movie.

The following day before the doctors came, Hermeline prayed and sang with me. The doctors pushed the chemo out for one more day. I hoped not to respond to it in the wrong way. My cousin took my mom on a city walking tour to take a break.

A peripherally inserted central catheter (PICC), also called a PICC line, is a long, thin tube that's inserted through a vein in your arm and passed through to the more prominent veins near your heart. Very rarely, the PICC line may be placed in your leg. A PICC line gives your doctor access to the large central veins near the heart. It's generally used to provide medications or liquid nutrition. A PICC line can help avoid the pain of frequent needle sticks and reduce the risk of irritation to the smaller veins in your arms. A PICC line requires meticulous care and monitoring for complications, including infection and blood clots-- Mayo Clinic Website.

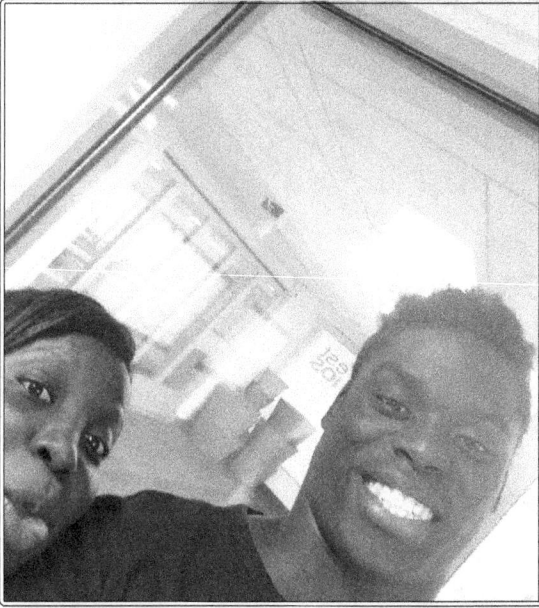

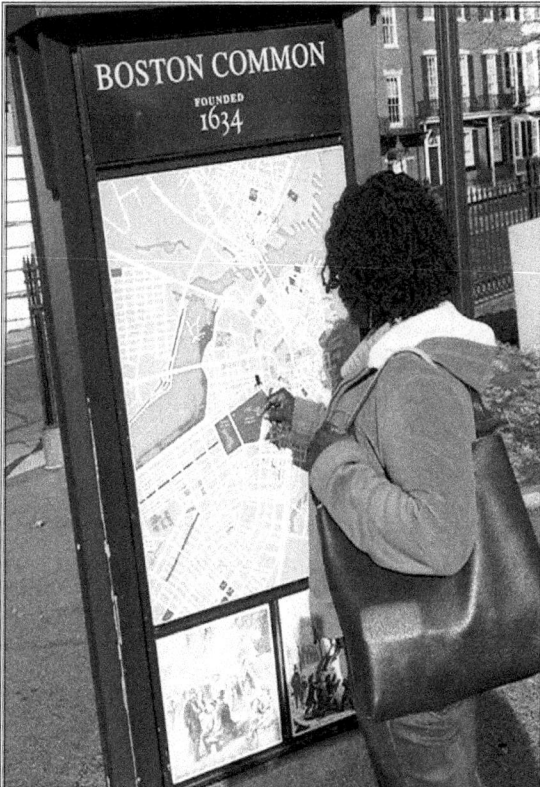

BOSTON COMMON
FOUNDED
1634

A positron emission tomography (PET) scan is an imaging test that can help reveal the metabolic or biochemical function of your tissues and organs. The PET scan uses a radioactive drug (tracer) to show both normal and abnormal metabolic activity. A PET scan can often detect the abnormal metabolism of the tracer in diseases before the disease shows up on other imaging tests, such as computerized tomography (CT) and magnetic resonance imaging (MRI). The tracer is most often injected into a vein within your hand or arm. The tracer will then collect into areas of your body that have higher levels of metabolic or biochemical activity, which often pinpoints the location of the disease. The PET images are typically combined with CT or MRI and are called PET-CT or PET-MRI scans.

--- Mayo Clinic Website.

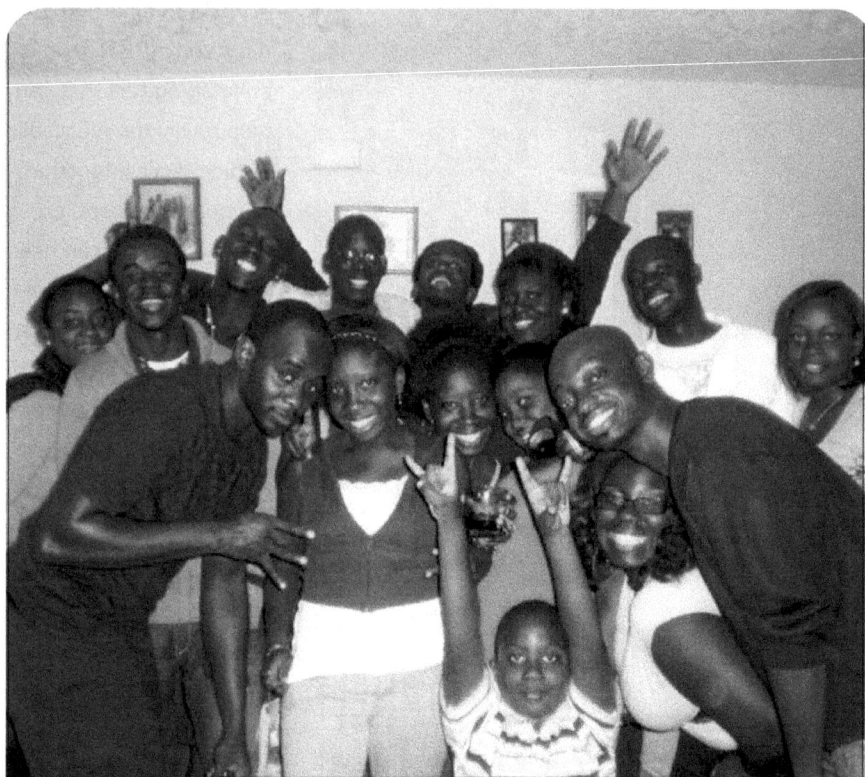

While they were gone, I watched Lost. Then I slept, ate, and made up my school assignments. I checked out Garage Band. It was not easy, but I could see myself getting better at it. Ironically as I was trying it out, my other cousin Sadrack called to check up on me. I happened to mention that I was using Garage Band. He has experience in it and gave me some tips. I also shared that I liked making music and producing my own. He sounded excited for me because he makes music as well. My other cousin Jephte also texted me. He is a fantastic rapper. I shared how I have been writing songs almost every day in the hospital, which he thought was great. After my conversation with Sadrack and Jephte, I felt that God revealed that I needed to make music with my family. I thought of writing a mixtape and putting something unique with my artistic family members.

I continued to enjoy my time alone. I listened to No Ceilings and But You Caint Use My Phone Mixtapes. I realized how unique music is and how one can create something appealing. I continued to write songs; many of them just came to me. Before my disease, I had writer's block and thought I had completely lost it. It is crazy how a dramatic change in life can produce good music. My mom says I find the good in everything. It can be hard to find happiness at the hospital, but I am doing well.

> It's crazy how a dramatic change can produce good music so out of someone.

As with everything, the holiday weekend ended, and Hermeline had to leave. The idea of her leaving upset me and made me realize how much I am stuck here at Boston Children's Hospital.

On day 9, I received a new chemo drug called Vincristine. I was expecting to feel terrible afterward, but everything was the same. It made the color of my pee look like grapefruit juice. I kept staying positive, and I started my English Exam. I saw that Luis, my friend who'd survived cancer, put out an E.P. with a song we wrote together through social media. I felt sad. My section of the songs was covered by someone else because I wasn't available. But after going through the emotions, I realized I have my special musical gift. I haven't had the chance to show it yet. I decided to learn the piano and explore my musical sound. I also felt guilty because I did not watch the Christ Fellowship online service as I would typically do on Sunday mornings. Also, I felt like I was using "the cancer card" to get stuff from my mom. For example, on Cyber Monday, my mom considered getting me a few things she had said no to before when I wasn't sick: a new T.V., desk, rug, and a MacBook Pro for my room. But ultimately, my mom bought me two hats, two beanies, jeans, and a sweatshirt—just $100 worth of clothes. Cancer was taking a lot out of me.

My mom felt terrible and brought me a few things to cheer me up.

On day 12, I started the last new drug. It sucked! I felt exhausted and experienced a lot of heartburn, which intensified throughout the day. I find it interesting that many bad things happen when I do not write in my journal. The nurse changed the dressing on my PICC line as I watched what seemed like an easy task. But my body did not respond very well from watching. I got very light-headed and had to lay down. I nearly passed out.

I binge-watched Lost. I did not finish my English essay as my energy was too low. My head was everywhere. I wondered: What am I or what will I do with my life? Will I ever find love? How will I be when I get home?

The next day, I lost my marbles. My mom asked if I would feel better if my sister Carmie was here? But of course, I did not see it like that. I felt like she did not like I wasn't engaging with her, so she proposed leaving and bringing my sister instead.

I am glad she is willing to do many things to make me happy, but I did not like it. Luis called, and we spoke for a good minute. He told me he does not know what he would have done without his mom when he was going through the same situation. I ultimately agreed with him. After the conversation, I apologized to my mom, told her how I felt, and hugged her. To me, her being here was enough. We made it up! You know how it is with mothers. They remember anything that strikes a chord in the heart, even if you fix it. I got some good news, too, as the doctors said I am doing well, my swollen lymph nodes are going down, and he advised that I kept doing what I was doing. By the end of the day, those deadly chest pains had finally stopped. I spent the rest of the day getting old pictures of my family members and friends, having epiphanies on the tile of the family mixtape. How about "Mind, Body and Soul" OR "Induction?"

My sister told me about a great recording session sale back at home. Patrick is getting better in music and theatre. I am proud of him but low-key; I am also jealous. I am not advancing in life because I am stuck here in Boston. But it is for the best. I know it. I need to follow my heart, stay focused, and be patient. Throughout my days at Boston, I find it interesting that many bad things happen when I do not write in my journal. So, I am going to try to keep up.

Chapter Three

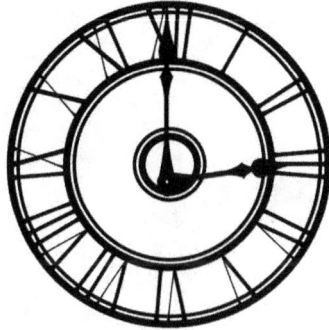

Surviving Boston Children Hospital
December 20, 2015 ~ Day 14-40

I have adapted to life at Boston Children's hospital. I was in a one-month drug cycle. I don't remember much after the first week, but I just know it was terrible. I took a new chemo drug every day along with steroids. The second week, I took one of the drugs from the first week. The third week, I took another chemo drug. It was during the third week that pancreatitis almost killed me.

My doctors gave me some good news that I could potentially be going home soon. I celebrated with a good breakfast (an amazing English muffin egg sandwich). I decided to have a good workout. My chest was pumping; my heart was beating hard. I felt invincible. Afterward, I took a well-deserved hot shower. It was going great at first, but it quickly turned bad. It appears my stimulating workout euphoric mood, along with the hot water and my medication,

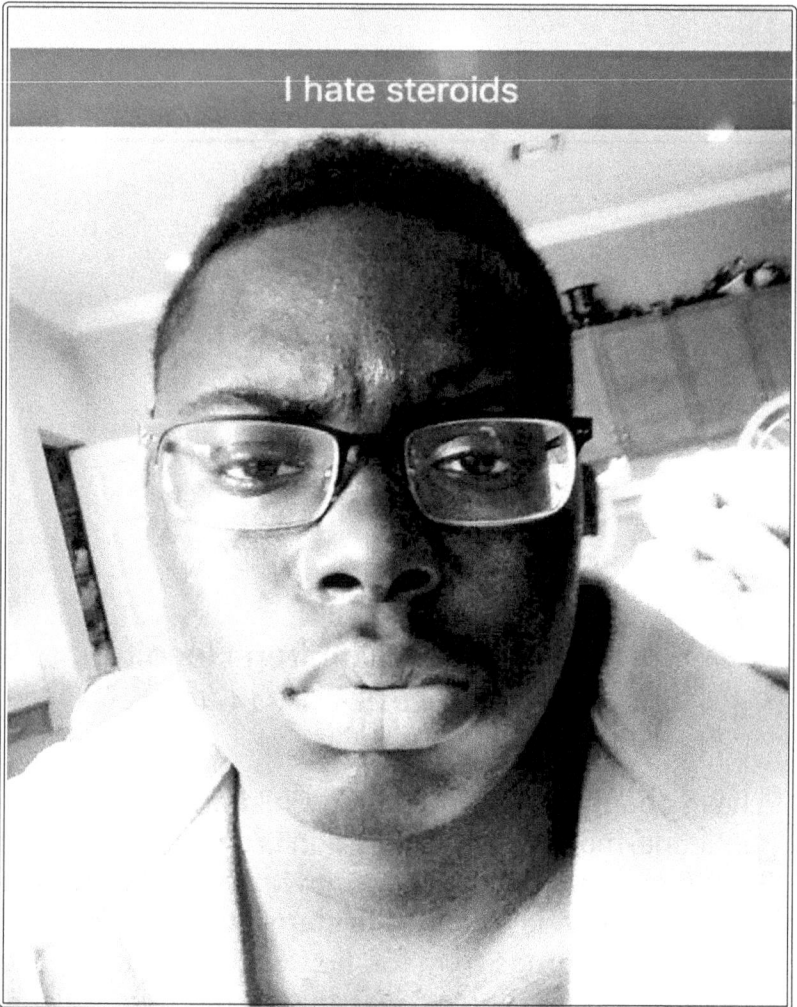

I hate steroids

were too overwhelming for my body. As a result, I nearly collapsed. It was terrible, my body was in pain everywhere, and I got the worst headache. I wobbled out of the shower, sat on the closed toilet seat, and tried to breathe, which didn't help. I started to see colors. My head was spinning. The steam from the hot shower was too much. I dried myself up, threw my clothes on, covered my tracks so my mom wouldn't notice, and collapsed on my bed. I slept for about an hour then came back to my senses. I told myself to man up and seized the day. My mom left to attend a parent painting session. I got out of bed, drank a liter of water, and ate half a sub. I figured moping around would not make me feel better and get me back to Florida to see my family and friends. So, I walked around with my mom when she returned. I did my homework and drank my 6 liters of required water intake. I once again seized the day by changing my perspectives. By late evening, I felt great again.

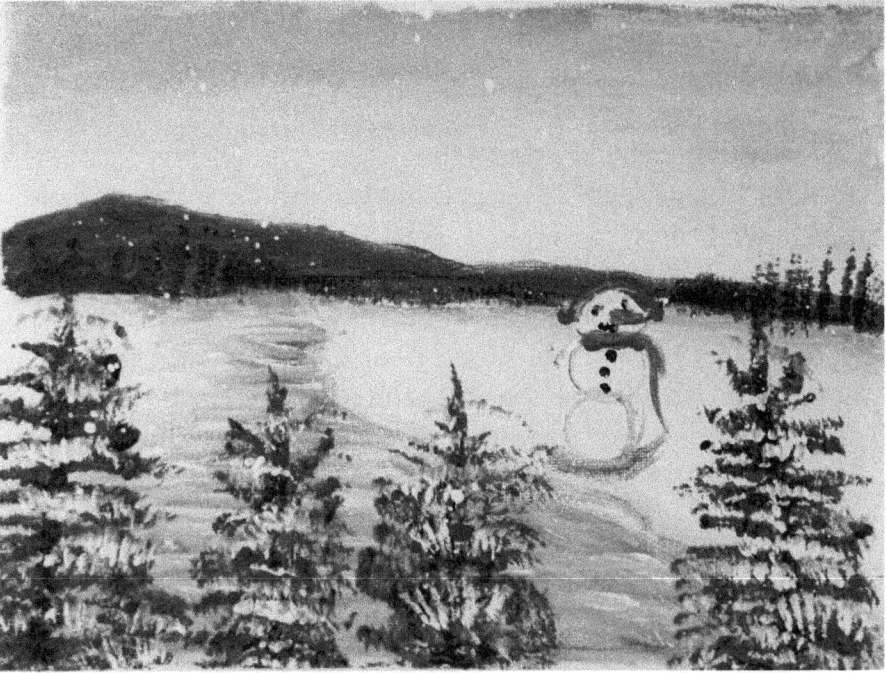

My mom painted the nicest Christmas picture At the parent painting session!

The day they took me off IV fluids, my dad relieved my mom. I was happy about his visit because he meant so much to me. Before my dad arrived, my mom and I visited the various gift shops in the hospital. My mom spent so much time looking at purses and bags in the gift shop. We tried a new and older cafeteria with the food we'd never tried before. We walked back to the hospital and had lunch there. I ate a six-inch Subway sandwich with chips, a side of fries, and a drink. After lunch, we went back to our room. Mom slept, and I finished my homework. I enjoyed spending this time with her. Even though she would only be gone for about a week, I knew I would miss her. After my homework, my dad called to let us know he was on his way. I was so excited to see him. It had been weeks. My dad walked in with slacks and a church shirt on. We showed him around and brought him to our room. He did not look as happy as I would imagine, but I know this is not easy for him.

After getting my dad situated, we went to the resource room for PIZZA NIGHT! I grabbed about three slices: cheese, meat lovers, and balsamic. I liked the balsamic pizza a lot because it was unique and different. Of course, I dunked on some cheese and sun chips on each slice. My parents did not eat too much but later got food near the hospital. It was nice seeing my dad. I know he is scared, but I wish he weren't. I am not afraid; I know God will help all of us. My dad had high hopes for me, his only son, as an athlete. Then all of this happened.

I had to start a legacy for this family. But what he does not know is that this is only making me and the people around me stronger. I know this is tough. My sisters say he is barely home anymore; he works long hours to cover all the bills. He has been doing this my whole life, starting with my private school, travel soccer, then my car, and now cancer. Before cancer, I planned to help my parents retire early. But now, God's willing, I plan to do a lot more than that. I hope I do not lose my marbles by then.

I went to bed late that night. The following day, I woke up at 7:30 a.m., and I felt like I only got 4 hours of sleep. Mom and dad were still asleep. A few people walked into my room, introducing themselves as my nurses. It was nothing but new faces, but I am thankful for any help.

My mom unpacked dad's luggage. My aunts send some extra clothes. I heard this clicking and clacking sound as my mom pulled out three soccer trophies and my high school diploma. My initial reaction wasn't the best. It was a grunt of disappointment. I mean, why should I be happy to see that stuff? I got bullied a lot through travel soccer. I did not get as much respect during high school soccer. Then on top of it, I did not get scouted for a good college.

It was cool being with my dad, though. I am glad we can hang out because he does not have much time to do that back home. We watched soccer and wrestling on the laptop. He told me about his old fighting stories back in Haiti. My dad and I watched Christ Fellowship, where a lady preached about hope-- passionate hope. She said you should count on it, pursue it, and expect it. My dad fell asleep, though. I love seeing my dad happy and enjoying himself, eating the foods he wants without second-guessing himself.

I had some great ideas about my music. I did not want to ruin it. It was crazy because I saw everything come together for once. I got Gabe, David, Patrick, Livy, Geo, and my cousin Sadrack to help with my E.P. My sisters are helping me brainstorm ways to use my experience to help other cancer patients. I got upset with them, though, because my older sister Nephtalie requested that I transfer money from mom's account to hers, which I had already transferred for my other sister Carmie to buy studio time. But Carmie did not. And the money went towards Nephtalie's bills instead.

After being away from home for about two weeks, word finally got out to everyone about my disease. A lot of my friends and extended family were in shock. They were praying for me and wishing me a speedy recovery. People donated to a GoFundMe account that my friend created. I saw God bless me in such a huge magnitude for the first time. It has God's writing all over it. I know he is planning something great for me.

I wonder what else he has planned...What am I, or what will I do with my life? Will I ever find love? How will I be when I get home? I do not know.... All I can do is keep praising him and let him do the work!

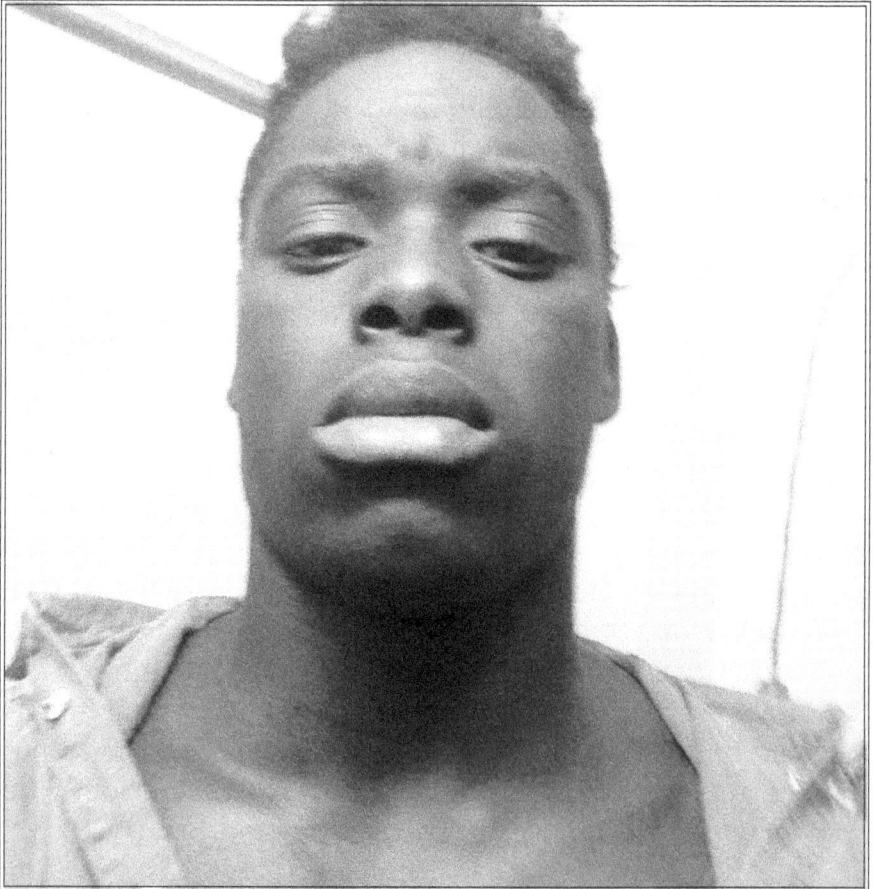

And today I realized it, and it has God written all over it. I know he's planning something great for me!

Being in a hospital setting for so long can be tiring. But a simple day without much happening is how you want your day to turn out. The routine is the same almost every day. Today was alright. I barely got any sleep last night. It was not easy to fall asleep. I rarely went into a deep sleep. I felt pretty good and confident because my lab results were good. The Chaplain stopped by and spoke to my parents for a while about her time in Haiti as a missionary. She asked if I wanted to share my story via a video series the hospital was doing. How could I say no to her? I agreed. Many people continued to give me support. I was surprised that even unexpected fellow players hit me up. I thought a lot of my soccer friends had moved on by now. I am glad a few of them checked in. It meant a lot to me.

I have not played the piano in two days, but I bond with my dad a lot. My parents paid for my next semester of college. I am so grateful for them. And to show that, I am thinking of using my GoFundMe® donations towards a vacation for them and studio time for me. They deserve it, and I do too.

Day 20 was a good day at the Boston Children's hospital. I woke up earlier than I usually did. I had my routine conversations with the chaplain. We talked about my essay, my special place, the pond where I live, and the Olympic Development Program (ODP) Wellington Wave Soccer Club that I played for. Before the video interview, the chaplain suggested that I accept a few visitors who were her friends. She introduced me, and one friend apologized for not coming by, which was cool with me. The others seemed nice as well. We even spoke about my favorite music genre and artist, Drake, since '06. I was surprised when one of them knew who Childish Gambino and Donald Grover were. I thought it was pretty dope that she had similar musical taste as me, and on top of it, she was cute.

I could not play music and hang with the Chaplain's friends because I had a full schedule. One of them offered to stop by later and help me record a song which made me extremely happy. She told me it is nothing fancy; it is simply a mic that she would set up in my room and connect to an existing software like Garage Band. I was probably cheesin like I was taking a picture. She could open a huge door for me without even realizing it. She also told me I could share my story and sing live on the Seacrest Studio. She confirmed that I could come back later after my cancer with my friends. Last week, she told me a patient admitted into the hospital six months ago came back and played Christmas music on the air. I wanted to explode with excitement hearing this.

All the puzzle pieces were coming together. Everything was looking good. I hope the rest of my days in Boston are like today. I pray for more days like this. I plan to finish my EP and play it on the radio with the people who helped me record it. That is my short-term dream. I can attain this dream. It is God who is doing all of this. It is so clear and vivid. I worried about the stomach acid that bothered me after I ate a taco and that my PICC line was about to get changed. I did not want to get light-headed again.

The next day, after having breakfast, stomach pains gripped me, leaving me bedbound for about two hours. After that, the physical therapist came in and asked if I wanted to go to the gym. I was not up to it, but I only get this opportunity once every two weeks. So, I laced up and went. My stomach was still hurting, but I was happy to have a gym schedule, even if it was limited. The gym was not really what I expected. I forgot I was at a children's hospital. But I was happy there was a treadmill. My P.T. watched me throughout my whole workout, which was uncomfortable, but he wanted to make sure I was ok. I walked quickly, but I could only jog for five minutes before getting exhausted. I was not even going that fast. It was kind of depressing because I was such a great athlete, and now I could barely jog. I was disappointed with myself, but there was nothing I could do. My stomach was hurting a lot, so I went to the bathroom and did what I had to do.

After that, I went back to bed. My stomach was still hurting, and I prayed for the pain to pass. I still think that Subway sandwich destroyed my insides, but it was completely worth it. I felt terrible to be in bed for so long because it was my dad's last day. I did not even play piano or walk around. My doctors said I was still improving and asked if I needed meds for the stomach pain. The stomach pain eventually went away without taking anything, which I was thankful for. I hope my dad enjoyed his time here. I certainly enjoyed spending time with him.

My dad woke up extra early to catch his 8 a.m. flight. While having breakfast that morning (he ate, I did not want to upset my stomach), he told me that he and my mom cried every night when they found out I had cancer. I also shared why I was emotional while I hugged him at the airport in Florida before leaving for Boston. I hugged my dad goodbye, went upstairs, and fell asleep while waiting for my hour-long Social Security Identification phone meeting scheduled for 9:30 a.m. They asked so many questions. My stomach was not doing too well from the cereal I had chowed down after my dad left. So, I went right to sleep after the meeting. I slept until around 11 am. I ate a delicious sub and ordered my food for the day: soup, salad, and mac and cheese. I ate all the food in about 3 hours. I could barely stay up to watch Christmas movies. During my nap, I had a wet dream. Going this long without any sex is challenging both mentally and physically. Usually, every part of me wants to masturbate, but I haven't.

The Chaplin came in to say thanks for doing the video and gave me the name of a person who wanted to help me create my blog. I never had so many people who wanted to check up on me before. But I did not want that right now because it was nice to be alone for once. I have not been on my own in two weeks.

My mom got some good Asian food and surprised me with egg rolls. The rice was amazing, but I liked the sushi a lot. The food was delicious. Later, we got soup, but it was not too fresh, so I did not like it.

I have surgery scheduled, and I need to finish my SLS project before Monday. My English essay and quiz are still due. I did not do too well on my quiz the first time, and I only turned in my rough draft for my essay. So, I have a lot of work to do. More and more people are finding out where I am and what is happening to me. Gabby has been very nice to me, and I cannot wait to be home so I can hang with her more. She is a fantastic friend and has comforted me a lot throughout this. However, I can't help but wonder if she is only nice to me because I have cancer.

Two of my friends are making an E.P. which I think is cool. I am happy for them, but I feel left out. I connect with them, and I think I should be there doing the E.P. with them.

After my last procedure, I got nothing but good news from the doctors. They told me that it was my last procedure at Boston Children's Hospital and that the final procedure scheduled for day 32 would most likely be done at home. And if I can stay healthy for the next 7-10 days, there is a possibility that I could go home sooner. All I have left is chemo and steroids treatment. That was wonderful news! I thanked everyone in the room for helping me. I gave mom my breakfast order from Dunkin' Donuts, and she delivered! I have not had Dunkin' in about two weeks, so I appreciated it very much.

My priority for the day was to finish my SLS project. One of the anesthesiologists offered to link me up with a healthcare administrator who would help me. The barber came around as she does every week to schedule patients for a haircut. So, I signed up. I am cutting it all off! I am ready. I am sure I will miss my hair, but one thing I do enjoy is to change. I want to do anything to make my mom happy. So, I also asked him about massages for patients' parents and requested that my mom be scheduled for one. We ordered three bowls of clam chowder for lunch and got bread from downstairs. I ate two bowls and saved one for later. My mom told me that she bought a new washer for the house and miscommunication with my sister. No one was home to open the gate for the delivery man. I tried to get them to realize it was a simply misunderstanding, but they are stubborn when they are "love hurt." After lunch, my mom got her nails done. I love it when she spoils herself. She does not do it enough.

But maybe I have something greater coming for me. Only God knows!

Finally, my sister Nephtalie helped me buy studio time online with her debit card since mine is inactive. It was pizza night, which made things 20 times better. We got our food but did not want to eat it yet. We walked around and looked for some water enhancers downstairs. We could not find any, but we found the crystal light powder, which was more than enough. I reached my goal of water intake for the day. When I got back, my nurse slid me a Gatorade Water Enhancer, which was nice of her.

My nurse brought in the Health Care Administrator to help with my SLS project. I recorded the entire discussion. She was extremely friendly and answered my questions. I did not start the project because the last bowl of soup put me to sleep for 45 minutes, and the Miami Heat game was on ESPN. I could barely stay up to watch it, though. I am thankful that my stomach pains are not as severe anymore, but my mouth sores worsen. Every third sentence, my mouth gets filled with saliva. The doctors said that it was normal.

Day 24 started very badly. I ate a full breakfast and ended up with a terrible stomach ache. I fell asleep on the couch for about an hour, then woke up to my aunt praying in Haitian Creole for me over the phone. I felt uncomfortable with lots of acid build-up. It gets more manageable when I open my mouth to burp. I have been spitting a lot more too, but at least I have no more mouth sores. I had obnoxious baby barfs, which I hate. For lunch, I ate a subway sub with chili. I wanted banana peppers and jalapeños, but I think those brought on these terrible stomach aches, so I avoided them this time around. I added guacamole, which tasted better, to make up for no spice. While eating, I watched the first episode of Season 5 of Lost. This show is so good! To remove the last round of chemo from my body and make up for my lost saliva, I was hooked to the IV for fluids on my walk with mom.

At this point, it was hard to envision going home. I could not believe my time here was almost done. The doctor said that I could be released within a few weeks. I happily shared the news with the nurses and told one of them, "I need to learn how to take care of myself when I get home!" I was so happy! It almost felt like I had not gone through anything. The nurse happily replied, "We'll go over that tomorrow." I needed to get a port in my chest that I did not want, but it would make life easier per the doctor's recommendation.

I sent a few of the family pictures to Carmie via email. She liked them. To me, everything was falling into place nicely. I was getting better. I have God to thank for all of it. I am finally going home!

So, I thought.

By day 34, a lot happened, and everything changed. I cannot remember it all. My mom filled in the blanks about what had happened to me over the past five days. The fact I do not remember is a good thing since it was so bad. I had a terrible reaction to some of the best-tasting lasagna I have ever had. My pancreas could not handle it, and it could have exploded. I was rushed to the Intensive Care Unit (ICU). I have been there before, but it could have been fatal this time. I remember being confused.

I started hallucinating about aliens coming to kill us. In my sleep, my mind told me that the light in the window was an alien; it went on to describe where it was born, where it lived, and how to defeat it. My mind told me that I was the only one who could stop the alien. So, the following day when the doctors came in to do rounds, I told them about the alien coming to kill us if we didn't kill it first. I looked and sounded crazy. I thought some lights in the mirror were indeed aliens. I started screaming and crying. I did not listen to the doctors or my parents. I thought people were throwing up, and I saw strange lights everywhere. I thought the evil doctor was killing my parents whenever they came to see me and stayed too long. I truly believed we were in grave danger.

I spent five days in ICU, which was not great, especially at night because I barely slept for three hours each night.

Let's face it; I was not ready for this.

Nothing felt the same when I woke up. I was on a regular diet, but I could not eat anything now. I would spit a hundred times a day. I could not use the bathroom, so I took many medications to manage my bowel movements. I have terrible diarrhea and go on my diaper twenty times a day. My mom or my nurse changed me, which was uncomfortable. I remembered one of the doctors standing outside the room while one of my nurses cleaned me. He never entered the room. I didn't think that was very nice of him. He was a mean doctor. Internally, I was a tad happy that he had to deal with my madness. But mostly, I was ashamed and apologetic to any doctor that came into my room during my hallucinations. I was embarrassed.

I lost my physical strength. I spent most of the days in ICU in bed. I slowly moved my legs, feet, and arms by day four. It hurt to stand longer than 10 seconds, and I almost fell when I tried. I could not walk. I wore my glasses for the first time in a week which helped a lot with the hallucinations. But they did not entirely go away until after a day or two. I felt a little taller, though, but very, very, skinny. I had a tube feeding me through my nose. A lot of tubes were in and out of me.

Oh, and brushing my teeth was the best feeling since I had not done it in a while. I was thankful not to remember most of those days. I remember a lot of what happened before the ICU, which had ups and downs. My mom had an altercation with my doctors, and my heart was getting bigger.

Unfortunately for my family and me, this happened around Day 37, which was Christmas 2015. Christmas Day marked my 37th day in Boston. Christmas was fantastic, not because I was home with family or because I received a significant number of gifts, but because Christmas eve was the first time I slept well in a long time. On Christmas Day, I walked a lot. I took a shower by myself and felt stronger. I watched every basketball game on T.V., and I was on a clear fluids diet. I took my melatonin medicine by mouth as it helped me sleep. I saw myself in the mirror. I wouldn't say I liked it, but I knew I needed to improve. I did not win the lottery, but I have more to be thankful for than money.

That feeling of contentment did not last long. I finally told Shela I had cancer, and she said to me that her dad got diagnosed after helping during 9/11, and one of her friend's mom was diagnosed as well. I felt overwhelmed and cried. I worried too much about my family. Being that it was Christmas, it made things worse. That night, I had a few hallucinations. I thought Nike signed me. I probably watched too much basketball. Then I had an opportunity to try a perfect drink (not sure how the two correlate). I also dreamt about baseball and how that could bring money. It was better than screaming or experiencing scary hallucinations while in the ICU.

Thankfully, the doctor promised to release me by New Years, if I kept improving. The following day, I woke up with more good news from the doctors; I continued to improve but needed to increase my water intake. I thought that was something I could easily accomplish. They asked for 4.5 liters, and I drank six by the end of the day.

I showered; it did not feel as good as the first time, but

that is expected. I had more clear chicken soup. I spent a lot of the day in my chair. I watched CNN and learned that eleven tornadoes swept through Dallas and left 50,000 people without power. Alabama was getting drenched with rain. I was worried about my friend J.D. and his family, but I learned they were not impacted. Europe is going crazy with the ISIS bombings. Mikey's family is from Italy, and he asked me about rice balls. So, I am having some when I get home.

The doctors advanced me on food today... Yeah! My mom and I had a long talk about family, and I know I can do a lot of good towards that. I texted my cousin Mardoshe. I do not want to have any missing links in the next generation of my family, my old church, family, friends, and cooking. Iyana tried video chatting with me, but I did not want to talk with anyone until I removed the feeding tube.

I walked about five laps and was able to move my legs and head without stumbling. I am preparing questions for my P.T. and doctors for departure. My mom and I are looking for flights. God blessed me. I almost died when I had pancreatitis, but I know God still has more planned for me. Today was a blessed day. Every day from here on will be like that.

MERRY CHRISTMAS!
I'm not done. Lol!
It gets A LOT
BETTER.

Chapter Four

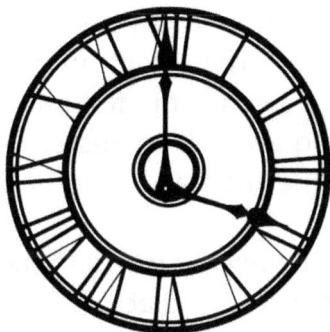

REGAINING A SENSE OF NORMALCY

New Year 2016 ~ Day 40-90 (Jan-April)

It was December 29, 2015, and we were about to ring in the New Year. That day, the doctors checked my cancer levels and told me that, unfortunately, I was not in remission. They also placed a port in my chest, which felt weird at first, but I got used to it throughout the day.

For the first time, I gave myself the blood thinner shot that I must get twice a day for six months because one of the chemo drugs gave me a blood clot in my left arm. I continued to get blood transfusions, especially when I was tired. It all left me feeling upset and scared.

My mom took it worse than I did. They offered me to stay in Boston, but we thought treatment in Miami was best—mostly to be closer to home. I told my mom everything happens for a reason, and God is in control. God has helped me so much along the way. I felt like I was missing out on a lot. I prayed and asked for things to go back to normal. Maybe this is the only place that could have brought me back after the pancreatitis incident. I know everything will be ok, so we need to keep fighting.

So, we started preparing to leave Boston and bought our tickets to fly home this week. Things were looking good. I broke the coffee machine trying to help my mom. I felt terrible. I am thankful that is all I was worried about that day. I signed up for online classes to start during the Fall semester because I thought it would be good for me mentally. God is doing good for me today.

God has helped me so much along the way!

The next day, I woke up needing more sleep. I ordered breakfast and ate it with my diabetic instructor. She taught me a lot about how to take care of myself. All the medical teams visited me every day for the last couple of days to get me ready to go home. So many people were coming in and out of the room every hour. Finally, mom and I had enough. On one of those days around mid-afternoon, mom and I were like, "OK... that's enough." We turned off all the lights, closed the blinds, and took our naps. Mom said it would work, but only if I went to sleep. And it worked! The only people who came in were my two leading doctors to give my mom some critical updates. After our nap, I ordered food again. Eating is a major problem for me. I am trying to gain weight, but I cannot raise my blood sugar. It's apparent, but I am confident I will gain the weight back soon.

I received more training for diabetes. I am eating better the more my confidence grows, and it feels great. I texted my family and friends to tell them that I could not wait to be home.

God planned for this, God will get me through this, and God has a reward for me when I win this battle.

Dec 31, 2015 - Departure 1 stop	Total travel time:5 h 43 m	
Boston	Washington	1 h 41 m
BOS	DCA	
1:00pm	2:41pm	
Terminal B	Terminal C	
American Airlines 2129		
Economy / Coach (Q) | Confirm seats with the airline *		
	Layover: 1 h 24 m	
Washington	West Palm Beach	2 h 38 m
DCA	**PBI**	
4:05pm	**6:43pm**	
Terminal C		
American Airlines 1741		
Economy / Coach (Q) | Confirm seats with the airline *		

I'm so ready to go home,
or I'll blow!
- Lyrics "Medications"
Jethro R. Pierre

By day 43 (December 31, 2015), I was home writing in my journal. But coming home from Boston was nothing like I expected it to be. I thought everything would go back to normal. I was wrong. My friends came over once a week if they were not sick because my immune system was too vulnerable to be exposed to any viruses. Family members and church visitors were in and out of my house. I could not play with my dogs Squanto and Lickie because I was too weak, and they could get me sick.

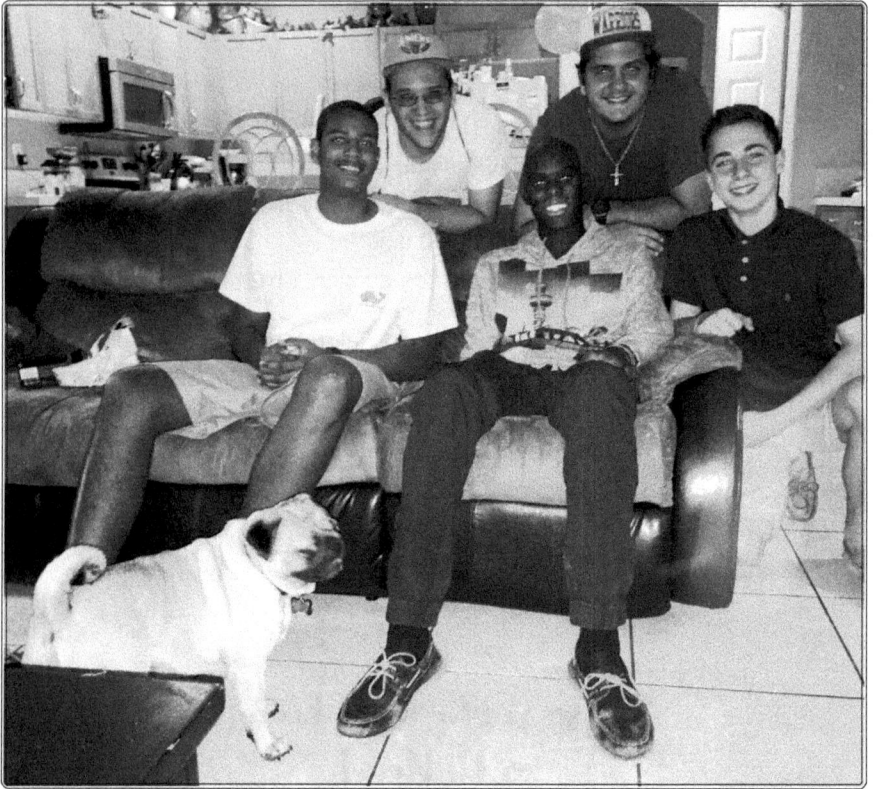

From left: Jordan, Mikey, Jethro, Brandon, Matthew
and Squanto!

I lost about 40 pounds in the ICU; I was bone thin. I could not fit in any of my clothes. The clothes my mom got me on Black Friday did not fit me anymore. My mom was terrified and forced me to eat as much food as possible. I get tired if I stand for too long. My mom and my sisters helped me with my showers. I avoided stairs as they were my worst enemy. My room is upstairs, so I brought everything I needed for the day downstairs so I wouldn't have to go back up until bed every morning. I would eat and watch television. I checked my blood sugar levels by finger pricking myself before every meal as I was diabetic. This took away my appetite. If my sugar turned out to be high, I took an insulin shot. By then, I was not hungry anymore. I did not drink anything with a lot of sugar, mostly water, crystal light, and milk, so my blood sugar would not increase. I took a whole bunch of pills.

My friends and I quickly realized I had amnesia. It was probably a side effect from my stay in the ICU and all the chemo because I could not recall some facts about our lives.

The first week of being home, my temperature was high, so I went to Palms West Hospital. I did not even feel sick, but I knew I had to go because I am susceptible to infection when my white blood cells are low.

A doctor must prescribe my medications because I am a cancer patient. I could not take Advil® or Mucinex® to help with my fever. When we got to the hospital, I was angry. I gave everyone an attitude. As usual, admission took forever, and I was in a small cold room for about two hours with my sister and dad. When our room was finally ready, they took me up to my bed. As we were going through the hospital, it all looked so familiar when I visited Mr. Houchins, who was admitted there before I got cancer.

I am ready to conquer life; the next, I am admitted for nearly a week. It is crazy how quickly life can change. I could not handle the truth and started to tear up. I was in the hospital for about six days. They kept me a lot longer than I thought they would. We thought they just wanted to bill more days. The last night I was there, I was with my two sisters. I do not know how we got into this conversation, but they noticed I looked depressed and wanted to cry. I was still caught up on how different my life was. I told them I did not want to cry in front of them, so I asked them to step out for a moment so I could gather myself. Once they left, I did not call; I wept. I wept because of how different my life was. I could not even recognize myself in the mirror. In my eyes, I saw defeat. I was in the room crying and simply yelling the name of Jesus. My mom told me when you are down and do not know what to do, merely say, Jesus. I was doing this for about five minutes before telling my sisters to come back in. Sometimes you must let it all out to move on from it, or you will remain stuck. The next day they discharged me. I was determined to get out of this, stay at home, and do nothing all day.

> My mom told me that when you are down and do not know what to do, just call on the name of "Jesus".

I gave myself the blood thinner shots. Mentally that is something challenging to do. Luckily, my mom is a well-experienced nurse; and my sister Nephtalie is a nursing student. Before work or school, I would get my first shot in the mornings, and once they arrived home, I'd get my second shot. They did my laundry, put my clothes away, cleaned the house, and took care of the dogs. I enjoyed not doing any of these chores, but I felt like I was becoming a burden.

As a very dependent person, I am not used to sitting around and having people do stuff for me. The first two weeks back at home after both hospital stays; I became comfortable and enjoyed spending time with my dad and sisters. My mom was working a lot more. It was challenging adapting without her. I am so used to her telling me what to do, and now I must figure everything out on my own. She would get home from work, and I wouldn't even say hi. I did not realize my actions, but my sisters did. I spoke to my mom about what was happening. It was a tricky situation for both of us. I tried to fix things too quickly, but she said she wanted to give me some space to grow.

I finally felt normal. I was happy to no longer be in hospitals and wanted to start living like a normal person again. I had to wear a mask in public when my blood counts were low and use hand sanitizer after touching anything. I went to my old high school and visited Mr. Houchins with my friends and Carmie. I enjoyed my first couple of weeks at home for the short time I was there.

Every Tuesday, I went to the clinic to check my blood to see if I was ready for more chemo. Unfortunately, during one of those visits, I learned I had to be on a new medical treatment which meant being admitted into another hospital— Holtz Children's Hospital in Miami for 11 days. Since I did not reach remission in Boston, I had to take harder chemo drugs. My cancer level was at 30% in Boston. To be in remission, I needed to be at 1%. I was at 3%. After those 11 days, I would stay home and recover for 3-4 weeks and then go in for another 11 days. I have a strong, stubborn cancer.

Encouraging others helped me.

I was admitted to Holtz Children's Hospital in late January 2016. My mom and I noticed that our room had two beds and was much smaller than Boston's. I did not want to get used to this, but I had no choice.

Ever since being in ICU, I could easily relate to other people's pain. I remembered hearing people crying, and I would cry too. I wanted to help them make their lives a little better. A girl in a room next to mine cried hysterically the day I left the ICU. I went to my room and asked my nurse to give her one of my teddy bears. I believed this could go a long way. The bear did not mean too much to me now but could mean a lot to her.

In Miami, my first roommate was a toddler. The first night, the toddler cried, and I started to tear up. That baby was going through a lot of pain, and I could relate. The nurse

47

explained the following day that they could not keep me in a room with a toddler because it is harder on the patient, so I moved two rooms down. I got a new roommate. He was my age but did not speak English. He needed assistance to walk. It was sad. It brought me back to Boston when I could not walk and spent my days in bed.

One night, when he was outside our room to practice walking with the P.T., I went for a bit of a walk myself. It is easy to get stiff and body cramps by staying in bed all day on chemo. I did two laps and went back to my room. As I walked into the room, I felt pushed to say something inspiring to him. I told him I related to everything he was going through. My PT trainer, who was bilingual, translated for me. I shared with them that I knew what he was going through. A few weeks ago, I could not walk either, now look at me. I promised him that it would not last forever. I told him he would get better.

The last four days of my first cycle in Miami did not end very well. I threw up everything I ate and drank. I went on myself plenty of times because my bowels were loose. I also peed on myself because I was on high fluids to get these harsh drugs out of my body. After each cycle, the side effects decreased.

My mom spoke with Luis' mom and learned that Luis did not reach remission after his first month of chemo either. He received treatment and achieved remission at Holtz too. I find it crazy how much Luis' journey is like mine. He had the same blood cancer as me. We live across the lake in the same neighborhood. My mom and I thought there were too many coincidences, and I am sure Luis and his family would agree.

I was discharged a day before my birthday! My family planned a party, and my friends helped. The party was fun; many of my family and friends were there, although I was too weak to enjoy it. When I saw Luis at the party, I hugged him and nearly cried. He said I was looking good and was surprised I still had my eyebrows. He said he looked a lot worse when he went through this, and I should be fine. Before he left, he told me that one of the hardest things to adapt to when going through this is not to date if you want to. I did not get it then, but today I do.

Later that night, I spoke with Shela. It was nice to see her. The last time I saw her was at a birthday party I was supposed to perform. I never did, but we all danced the whole night. She called me her dance partner. Although she was happy to see me, I noticed she was not in the best of spirits, so I asked about her father. She was not feeling too good and needed someone to speak to, especially after her grandfather passed. I related to how she felt and wanted to give her a teddy bear as I did for that girl in ICU.

Towards the end of the party, I got lit. Carmie brought down my Xbox. Skyler brought his Xbox over from his house, and Jordan brought his speakers. Matthew was the DJ, and he danced around like the hype man he was. Skyler was with Elizabeth, JD did not talk to his girlfriend the whole night, and we roasted him for that. Mikey was playing Xbox with Jordan. Gabe, Alex, Garfield, David, and I took pictures on Lisa's dope camera. Gabby, Lauren, Iyana, Azyah, Diana, and Vicky were dancing and singing along with Matthew. When I got to the cake to blow it, everyone said I looked upset. They didn't realize that I felt truly blessed to have some of the most incredible friends in the world. I looked down at the cake, looked up, smiled, and blew out the candles. It was a fantastic night. It felt good to be 19.

Superbowl Sunday ~ February 2016

The weekend came, and it was Super Bowl Sunday. I did not care much for it because I'm not a big fan of American football. The only "football" I know is "Soccer." But I was excited because my chorus friends—The Squad— made plans to watch it at Iyana's house. I was ready for football, commercials, snacks, and spending time with my friends. I could have even gotten sick as a few people came to the party ill and did not tell me until the end. I did not want anyone to feel bad, so I told everyone I was fine, even though I knew I would be sick in a few days.

However, we had a big argument because a few friends from the Squad made their own plans. Matthew invited the guys to Sonny's house to turn up. I did not see the fun in that. A whole bunch of dudes are turning up. I rather have fun with "The Squad" at Iyana's house.

I left my house upset. Jordan and Matthew decided to go to Sonny's, so I went to Walmart by myself. I got snacks and a gallon of juice. I struggled to carry it to my car; it was embarrassing, and I finally drove to Iyana's house. It was a lovely night with those who were there. We had fun, and we chilled. It was lit.

The ride home from Iyana's house was amazing. It felt like I was back in October of 2015, back when things were normal. The music was loud; I was singing. The road was clear with no traffic. I live for these days.

The next day, my friends and I laughed about the arguments over the super bowl party and roasted each other about it in our group chat. And life went on.

Super Tuesday rolled around, and I was admitted again. I did not have a roommate this time, which was nice. I spent the first two days catching up on my Dragon Ball Z. Then, I finally got sick from all the Super Bowl germs. Being sick felt worse because I was on chemo. It is a terrible combination. I was coughing and had a lot of mucus. I was throwing up. It was horrible. To help, the doctors gave me antibiotics, but my dad kept giving me tea with honey as if I was a normal child.

Before I was admitted again, they checked my Bone Marrow Aspiration to confirm I was at .01%, which would mean that we could start the Bone Marrow transplant. Instead of being at .01%, I was at .02%. It sucked, and I immediately felt depressed about it. I threw on my headphones, turned on Ultralight Beam, and let the tears roll down my face as I stared at the ceiling. I did not eat breakfast because I most likely would throw it up. I felt like I had run out of answers. I did not know what to do.

That night I had the worst nightmare. It was a lucid dream. I jolted out of bed in the middle of the night. My pants were wet. I started freaking out, and my mom was scared. I began to cry and kept telling her they were coming to kill me. I threw off my clothes and exposed myself to her. Maybe we still had some time to getaway. She went along with what I was saying so she could calm me down. I kept crying and told her the nurse would kill me for wetting the bed. She held me and told me that wasn't true. She got in my bed and comforted me. She told me it was nothing but a bad nightmare. She told me the devil was trying to get to me. It still didn't make me feel any better.

The nurse came in, and I was frightened. My mom told me, "she isn't here to hurt you." I asked the nurse if she would ever hurt me. She said no, and my fear changed to sadness. The nurse and my mom comforted me. I asked the nurse if she believed in God. I wondered if I could hold her hand, and then we all prayed. My mom slept in my bed that night. It turned out that the nightmare I had was like that awful hallucination I had in Boston. It was a terrible nightmare.

I felt down the following day. My psychiatrist came in, and we spoke about my dream. It is always nice talking to him, but I remained in a low mood the whole day. I could not eat. I wanted these 11 days to zoom by. I went to bed early, simply hoping for my days to end. I kept falling in and out of sleep. I had body pains everywhere, and I was very uncomfortable. When I fell asleep, I had the craziest and most apparent dreams. Throughout all this sadness and sickness, I managed to think about Elizabeth Marie.

A Sigh of Relief ~ March 25, 2016

After my first cycle, I reached remission! I went from 3% to 0.7%. I started to drive again. I got a new laptop. I saw my friends and cousins more often. I cleaned my room and took showers by myself. I stayed out longer, and I was not on the couch as much. My mom and I went to a support group meeting with the Pediatric Oncology Support Team (POST), supporting cancer patients and their families in South Florida. We met some lovely people there. They understood our situation and told us if there was anything we needed, do not hesitate to ask. I asked for an Xbox. I told them it could come in handy when I am in the hospital and cannot talk to my friends. This way, I can still interact and play with them.

The Pediatric Oncology Support Team (POST) helps local children and their families (in 6 South Florida counties) courageously fight cancer by giving them compassionate emotional and financial support. We partner with families to provide support, teach new skills, offer new perspectives, and help to reinforce their natural resiliency.
Visit www.postfl.org to learn more.

Then a week later, an Xbox was sent to my house! We sent a thank you letter. POST does more than giving free stuff, though. They listened to my story and found ways could help our family financially, physically, and emotionally. It is a great organization, and they will do whatever they can to help a family fighting cancer in South Florida.

I relied on my sister Carmie so much since being home. She is home with me most days. In the mornings, she makes whatever I want for breakfast... it's great! I wish more people had siblings like her. We hung out with Mikey and went to my cousin Mardoshe's high school basketball game. I saw my uncle and all my other cousins as well. It is fantastic to see how much they have all grown up. I truly wish nothing but the best for them all.

I did not realize how much I missed everything until I got to experience it all over again.

It was another Tuesday, so I went for another weekly check-up at the clinic in Miami. They ran blood tests, weighed me (I was not gaining any weight despite how much I ate), checked my vitals, height, and temperature—all the usual stuff. My main oncologist gave me some pressing news. Since my cancer was at its lowest, it was time to decide on the Bone Marrow transplant.

I was terrified and wanted to say no. He told me that cancer would most likely come back if we did not do the transplant. He advised that they check my sister's first to see if she was a match. Soon after, we met with a Bone Marrow Specialist. She told me that Bone Marrow treatment lasted four to six weeks because I needed to be carefully examined throughout the process to get a new host in my body. She explained that my body could reject the transplant.

I was not wholly comfortable with this yet. I figured it would take some time for it to all sink in.

A bone marrow transplant is a procedure that infuses healthy blood-forming stem cells into your body to replace your damaged or diseased bone marrow. A bone marrow transplant is also called a stem cell transplant. You might need a bone marrow transplant if your bone marrow stops working and does not produce enough healthy blood cells. Bone marrow transplants may use cells from your own body (autologous transplant) or a donor (allogeneic transplant).

- The Mayo Clinic -

Chapter Five

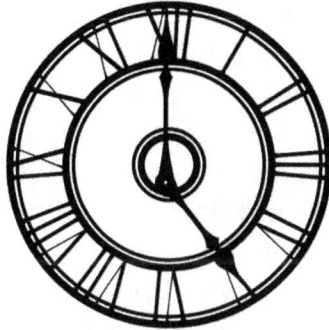

Bone Marrow Transplant
April 2016 ~ Day 0

On April 18, 2016, I was admitted to the Sylvester Comprehensive Cancer Center in Miami for a bone marrow transplant. Over time, through several tests, they found a donor, a DNA donor, my sister Carmie. Because she is a DNA donor, the recovery period would be quicker and less complicated. It is still a very invasive procedure with multiple side effects. New cancer could develop; there could be a lesser chance of having kids, and I could die from the infection. I have faced death before. I can tell you it is not fun. To be able to walk away (or wheel away) from what happened to me in Boston was a blessing.

My nurse asked if I had a living will. People ask me this question often, and the answer is always "No. I'm too young for that." This whole thing stressed me out. I wasn't feeling suitable for a few days. I signed out of all my social media accounts. I did not text anyone. It was crazy. I was looking forward to a great vacation with family and friends this summer. I was getting ready to move on from this chapter in my life, but something always turned up.

I was scheduled to be in the hospital for three and a half weeks and then had to stay near the hospital for an additional three months. In the hospital unit, there were stringent rules— no outside food. I rarely went out in public. I wore a mask and gloves everywhere I went. I did not see my dogs the whole summer. My hair fell out again. I had several bad days, full of tears and fake smiles. It is hard to get used to all of this, but I found a way. I didn't have any choice. I would have if I did not see God's hands in all of this. I would have said "YOLO" and been on my way, not caring whether cancer returned or now. But the fact that I had a DNA donor who was an exact match and more than willing (no matter how much I bothered her as a little brother) were reasons enough to keep me going.

Radiation for the Bone Marrow transplant was intense. My sister got a Neupogen shot; she said it burned severely, and I got eight radiation treatments to kill my white blood cells before they could do the bone marrow transplant.

The nurse wheeled me downstairs with my mom by my side for the first time. I knew what to expect because we rehearsed it, but I still nearly passed out. The radiation took a while. I stood in this tight place for about 15 minutes. The doctors instructed me to not move while they drew on my body with a sharpie. At one point, it became way too much for me. I got light-headed and almost passed out from the anxiety. I sat on the chair, scared out of my mind. Not ready for any of this. It all seemed too much and was becoming too normal. I nearly cried, but I toughed it out and finished the radiation treatment without any interruptions.

My second radiation treatment was quicker but not without issues. The machine restarted again during my treatment and overheated. So, the wait was long, and I threw up in between treatments. I felt better after that, though. They fixed the problem, and I got everything done. I went back to my room with my mom, feeling entirely out of it. I ate lunch which did not sit too well. I watched a movie on Hulu and took a nap. My nap got interrupted about three times with people coming in to check up on me.

I am halfway done: four down, four more to go. In the waiting room, I stared into space. Nothing felt right in my body. The doctors and nurses said everything should go faster for the next two days. Since I got up this morning in a rush, I did not have time to change out of my pajamas. So, everything was hanging loose. I knew everyone could tell, but I could not do anything about it. All of this was funny but very embarrassing. But, hey, no shame, I am blessed.

> I am halfway done: four down, four more to go.

I did not do too much between my radiation treatments. I walked daily to keep my muscles strong. I tried to be as responsible as possible, so my mom wouldn't get on my back. On one of those days at radiation, I forgot to take one of my mouthwashes. After taking four types of mouthwash, one every two hours, I forgot one. I died inside because I knew my mom was getting ready to chew me out. She did it in front of the nurses, which I did not think was nice. We went back and forth at each other. I was tired of her coming at me the way she had lately, and she did not like that I was disrespectful. I pulled the "I am an adult…. I'm 19" card. I knew it was stupid to say, but I didn't care. I was pissed. The conversation didn't end too well, and I could not let it stay there. I apologized as I knew deep down it was my responsibility to take my medications. She should have been tougher on me, to be honest. Eventually, I got on top of my meds.

The hospital was boring, and I wanted some company. I wanted my friends. I thought, "I'm asking for too much. Some patients are on their own." My loving sister Carmie surprised me with a shirt she got at the OVO pop-up shop nine minutes away from the hospital. The shirt was an extra-large that was too big for me, so I planned to frame it and hang it up.

I learned from my mom that one of my favorite artists and inspirations, Prince, died (April 21, 2016). It was everywhere online and all over the news. I felt sad about his death because he inspired me and many others. He influenced people to know what they stand for, no matter what others think. When I was in Boston, I watched his 2008 Coachella performance, where he performed his song "Creep." I love the whole vibe and how he could completely take over an audience with his stage presence. I looked up to him when it came to be different. I was so into the moment that I started a beat that day.

During my radiation treatments, my mom and I bonded more. We spoke about my future girlfriend and how she needs to know how to cook (my mom planned to teach her if she did not know), my dad's dream of opening a restaurant, and future vacations we'd take as a family. It was nice to have conversations like this with my mom. My mom left for work while my sister stayed with me. I could not kiss her goodbye because I could not get sick.

The radiation worked fast. Some days, I had radiation twice a day for three days straight. The main side effect was that I threw up all the time. I could not keep anything in my stomach. I was getting a lot of mouthwashes and shots to help heal my mouth sores, so food did not taste the same. I was down about that. My Ramen Noodles tasted like metal! After multiple requests, my family brought me Baked Ziti, but it tasted bland. When I eventually regained my taste, the first thing I ate was Ramen Noodles and Stouffer's! I killed it!

I finished my radiation treatments. I got to ring a bell and say a poem to commemorate it. I was glad to be done with this first part because it was one of the hardest things I ever had to go through. Since I was not as scared or tense anymore, I signed back into my social media accounts and texted again.

I received another round of chemo right after radiation treatments. My nurse gave me an Ativan to help reduce my nausea. That drug is a sedative. I felt loopy, as if I was tipsy. I stayed in bed for an entire day. My aunt Lucie came by, but I slept the whole time. I felt bad. She understood because she's in the medical field. I woke up feeling terrible. I felt that at any moment, I could throw up. It sucked. That day she visited, I skipped breakfast and lunch. Luckily, Matthew, Mikey, and a few other friends called me and brought soup. This was all to make me feel better, which worked. I was glad to see them and ate about four bowls of soup that day. My oldest sister, Nephtalie, stopped by and took Carmie out for lunch. I was glad she got out because I knew it was a lot on her. As my older sister Nephtalie hugged me goodbye, I could tell she was scared like the rest of us.

My New birthday (April 18, 2016)

Although, I appreciate what my sister Carmie was about to do to give me another chance at life, I was stressed, scared and worried. It was finally Day 9 (the day of my Bone Marrow Stem Cell Transplant). I tried everything, including sleeping, to take my mind off my current situation. At this point, I was able to sleep, and I felt like I was in a different world. My world. A world without fear, stress, or worries. Then I wake up weak. I was barely holding on. To get some hope and look forward to the future, I made plans to see Drake in concert. It was a medal for all my efforts. I also watched the Heat game, which they lost ...so I was angry. I video chatted with friends and family who gave me early birthday wishes.

My new birthday went a lot better than expected. I have endured so much. I got hit with the Ultra-Light Beam (radiation) eight times in a row with one dose of chemo. I was ready for the transplant.

My mom came early to accompany Carmie while they extracted the stem cells. It was a six-hour procedure, but they had more than enough at the halfway point. While I waited, a lady came in and set up a piano in my room. She showed me how to play "Hold on We're Going home, Hotline Bling, and Marvin's Room." I think with more practice; I could nail these songs. She had experience with music production and taught me some tricks on Garage Band. I was excited as she planned to help me with a lot more in the future. My mom and sister returned and took naps on the pull-out bed together. I torched my dad in the FIFA game on my Xbox. I showed no mercy. It was fun playing with my old man. I knew he enjoyed it because he smiled and laughed the whole time. I love that no matter how hard times got, my family was always close by.

My nurse prepped me for the Bone Marrow Transplant. I fell asleep during that. THE PROCEDURE WAS OVER when I woke up, and I hadn't felt anything.

The most challenging time was the two weeks after my transplant, and my patience had never been tested so much. I could not leave until my blood counts had increased, which usually took 12 days or so. Around Day 3, my white blood cells count was .6, my hemoglobin was 7.6, and my platelets were 115. I was getting blood transfusions. I threw up daily. I was itchy on some parts of my body; it felt like a flame was being lit under the balls of my feet, and I had not eaten a complete meal in days.

On May 1st, Jordan's family visited. They have been a great support to me throughout all of this. They encouraged me to eat as I explained my loss of appetite. They are like my second family. I had many of those now because my friends' families treated me as if I were one of their own. My sister Carmie looked happier. I liked seeing her this way. She was about to get a promotion in her job. I was looking forward to seeing a lot more of her. My mom brought me some home-cooked rice and chicken. It did not taste the same because of the meds, but it was much better than the hospital food. Everyone was getting along, and the nurses were more excellent lately. It made my stay a lot better. My mom spoke with one of the nurses, who said that many firefighters were getting cancer and discovered that something in the uniforms was causing it. She went on to mention that turf grass athletes use is not safe. I played soccer countless times. I often wondered how this happened to me. Was it Squanto, Tori, or Vicky, the dust at my job, or even working out too much?

Days at the hospital continued to be boring. The Wifi was not great, so I could not play Xbox. I watched movies instead. I listened to Drake's new album, which was good. All my friends were out, having fun at Sunfest, clubs, and parties; they were enjoying the summer. It was hard to watch. I felt so isolated and far from home. I felt like I was in prison— the visits, the foods, and talking about plans that probably would not happen. I was entirely out of my comfort zone. I cannot stress it enough; it was terrible. My facial expression shows how much I was done. Everyone could see it. I could not help it. I wanted it to end. I cried the first time since being admitted. This was hard on me. I was missing out on so much. It was hard to deal with. I was gone from friends, and I was so weak at the same time. I was itching for comfort, and I wasn't getting it. I made a promise to myself that when I got out, I would make up for the lost time. I deserved it. I had been through some tough stuff. The only way I got through it all was by reading the word of God, but I was not able to do that. I was so disappointed in myself. I had the answer right in front of me, and I neglected it. I was not doing anything better with my time. I was just sitting around. When I applied to a Make-A-Wish for adults called "3 Little Birds 4 life," I was asked, "What would be a Perfect Day or Experience for you?" I spent several days contemplating this question. I could not decide. There is so much I want to do, but I can only choose one. At first thought about going to OVO FEST (Drake's three-day music festival with notable celebrities and Canadian artists in Toronto, Canada). I could go with some friends and meet Drake, but what about my family? It would be hard to travel that far with my friends. Then, I thought I should spend a weekend with family and friends in Disney World and stay in the castle for a night. It would be too hard to prepare, and few people would go. I shared many of these ideas with the people I love. They think I should do what I want to do; I deserve it. I know I have gone through a lot, but they deserve something just as much as I do. I have learned throughout this journey that cancer not only affects me; it affects everyone around me that I know and love. Then I settled on this answer "A Perfect Day would be a Book Launch Party with all my friends, family, cancer survivors, and a Drake performance. That would be the Perfect Day for me. I could not think of any other way to put an end to all of this." I hope they get back to me. I am very excited! That would be the Perfect Day for me.

As I approached Day 12 after the transplant, everyone tried to boost me up, get me to eat food, and encourage me to walk. My body was not cooperating. I know how much of a pain I can be to other people. It was like there were two parts of me—one that was dying and falling apart and the other watching and hating every minute of it. Honestly, I do not know how long I will last before I completely snap. I was angry and felt like I had no control over this situation.

One morning, my nurse told me, "May the force be with you," as I got out of bed. I'd never felt so fatigue and tired my whole life. My platelets were very low (6); it showed in my body. I had never been so scared either. There was blood in my stool and urine. It freaked me out. But my mom said it was expected when the platelets decreased. I took a shower, but my body could not even handle doing that. I couldn't even finish my walk. I got back to the room and threw up half of my breakfast. At this point, I was done with the day. My doctor ordered a platelet transplant. I tried to relax for the rest of the day. My mom left for work, and my sister and dad came soon.

I spent Mother's Day away from my mom because she had to work. Carmie and I had a deep conversation about family, friends, the future, and relationships. She wanted to know why I hadn't gotten with a specific girl, but I told her the timing was not right.

I was in a lot of pain from the Neupogen shots. It felt like someone had put their heel in my back and was applying severe pressure on it. I took an Ativan and a sleeping pill, and Oxycodone. The pain was so much that I wanted to cry. It was the first time I had taken a severe pain medication like Oxycodone throughout all of this.

I was hoping to leave the hospital on May 10, but the doctors were worried that I was not eating enough and that my kidneys were not doing too well, so they kept me longer. My mom was mad at me because she felt I was not pushing myself enough. She was on my back to walk and drink more water. I was off the Caphosol mouth rinse, and my taste buds had returned to normal. My mom brought me a taco, and I ate it in seconds. Patrick asked me to perform a song with him at Iyana's Graduation party. I was hesitant but agreed because Iyana is special to me. I would do anything to make her happy. Also, I wanted to do something with Patrick.

The Ronald McDonald House ~ May 2016

On May 13, after three weeks of being at Sylvester, the doctors finally agreed to discharge me to the Ronald McDonald House, where I stayed for another three months. They gave me a booklet with a questionnaire to ensure I knew how to take care of myself after being discharged. I got every question right, but one. My mom did not feel comfortable with me leaving the hospital yet, mostly because she wanted to be the one to help me settle at the Ronald McDonald House.

But thankfully, my sister convinced her to let me leave. She promised we would be careful and that she would make sure I wore my mask and gloves, not eat fast foods, and take my meds. My mom wanted to call off work, but we would not let that happen because we had bills. As I was getting discharged, my nurse, who was pregnant, complimented my family because she said that I was one of her politest patients. She promised to pray for me. I promised to pray that she delivered a beautiful baby.

As I walked there, my sister and aunt brought my stuff to the Ronald McDonald House which was right next to the hospital. It was easy at first, but my feet began to burn as I got closer. It felt like I was walking on hot coals. It was terrible. I have not felt this in a while. We finally arrived at our room where my sister and I settled. The move went well.

The house had its ups and downs, but it was better than being in the hospital. Eventually, I felt better. I stopped throwing up. I took my meds and ate well. Despite how annoying I was, my sister Carmie took care of me, and I appreciated all her hard work. My mom was impressed with my improvement. I met with the nurse practitioner, who was incredibly lovely during my check-up. We talked about careers. She said my kidney levels are high, and I need to hydrate more. I could feel my mom scolding me with her eyes. I stayed longer to get fluids. I asked my Nurse Practitioner permission to go to Wynwood with my friends. I told her I needed to do something, or I was going to go crazy. However, she said that it was too soon. My heart sunk, and everything she told me after that went in through one ear and out the other. My mom would not let me go since she knew how risky it was. I told my friends, and only Patrick responded. I was down about it. What was I supposed to do in Miami for three months? Stare at the wall? That is what I did. My TV at the Ronald McDonald House barely worked. We got 15 English channels and 100 Spanish channels. I was worried I would not celebrate any of my friends' graduations with all these restrictions. I caught up on much-needed sleep; I visited Publix and Walmart with my mom. It was nice being out, although I did not do much. At night, I played XBOX and talked to my friends.

After visiting home, my sister Nephtalie drove me back to the Ronald McDonald House, and Carmie met us later. I was happy because I got to be with my family, friends, and dogs Squanto and Lickie! I hung out with both of my sisters. My younger sister Carmie wasn't too happy that we didn't do much.

I was depressed because my doctor would not let me go to my friend's graduation or attend graduation parties. Whenever I opened Snapchat, I saw everyone having fun without me. Parties at home, bottles everywhere, and people were dancing. It killed me to miss out on that.

I thought I felt a small lymph node behind my ear. But if the same thing happened again (which I prayed it wouldn't), I would be destroyed physically and mentally. I could not go through more treatment.

Radiation made me darker, the transplant affected my walking, and I had more fat. I could not even go for a girl. To be honest, who would even want to be with me? If anything, it would be for sheer pity. I felt hurt. Even though I could work out, did I even want to? I could barely put a homemade taco together without getting out of breath. It was hard to do it again! Was it wrong to ask why me? My life was so great back in the day. I hated myself for not realizing it then. It was probably why I got it taken away from me. I did not appreciate it the way I was supposed to. I would do anything to go back to it. I found my student ID from college. I stared at the old me, so young and innocent. He did not know what was coming in a few months. There was nothing he could have done to stop cancer from happening.

Chapter Six

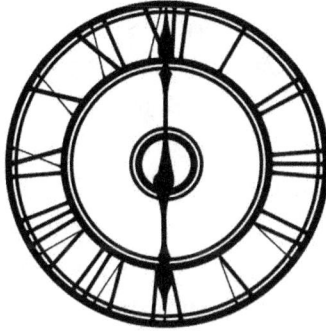

Reconnecting with The Squad
Summer 2016

In early June, my doctor cleared me to work out and go back to school. I was confident that I would leave within a few days. As an independent person, it feels great to go back to some sense of normal.

At the Ronald McDonald House, a new family from Hawaii moved in next door to us with a boy around my age with Acute Myeloid Leukemia (AML). He had heart failure while going through treatment and almost died. Because of our similar journey, our moms instantly connected. They spoke daily and exchanged stories during their pedicures and manicures. I felt his pain because I relate to how different his life was. He was tall and skinny like me. He used to play basketball. Now, he had appointments every day at the hospital. His AML came back after he was cured. I could only imagine how he must have felt. There were two scared boys on both sides of this wall. I prayed for his heart to be healed after his heart failure like my pancreas healed after my Pancreatitis.

On June 11, 2016, my doctor discharged me! My labs were terrific, and the doctor did not think I needed another blood transfusion. Unfortunately, I got one a few weeks later. I was thrilled to be home for good. I missed my bed, Squanto, family, and friends. My parents were strict with me, though, especially my dad. He did not want to see me end up back in the hospital because I was foolish.

I felt better. My hair was growing soft and curly. I got a college scholarship. I spent a lot of time with my friends playing Xbox games: Run Escape, Pokémon Go, Halo Combat Evolution, and FIFA (soccer). Matthew, Tim, and I went to the mall to pick up birthday presents for my sisters. My sister Nephtalie was graduating from Nursing School. I cleaned my room and made music, and I was proud of my progress in producing beats. I started Music Mondays. I released a new song with attractive cover art every Monday. I was excited to be doing this series. It showed people what I could do as an artist. Matthew and I were also working on new projects together.

During the summer, most of my friends went on vacation. Matthew went to Italy for a week. He got me an Italian hat, a map of Italy, and a book of butts; yes! A book of butts. He got Mikey's birthday present as well. I could not wait until August to eat out and do what I wanted, except swimming, which was still out of the question. My family was planning a very much-needed vacation. I do not look like a stick anymore, but I am still fragile. Matthew joked about that, but I told him, "You're here laughing instead of in the gym preparing for my full-fledge come back. You're not ready." No one was ready. Honestly, I do not know if I was prepared because it was not easy to jog. I was exhausted, and my feet felt heavy. My blood count continues to increase. The doctor tapered down my Tacrolimus (an immunosuppressive drug), suitable for my kidneys.

In early July, my doctor ordered a Bone Marrow Aspiration to check for any sign of cancer. It was uncomfortable. As they drilled in my back, I felt a shock around my left leg. Other than that, I recovered quickly. Since I was doing so well, my doctor removed the Trifusion Port from my chest. It felt weird. I was wide awake and was not sedated. I felt very free after they removed it!

I was excited to get my life back on track, play sports, eat the food I wanted, and get back to school, work and be with my friends. I tried to find someone and date. I tried to put myself out there again. I could go to the gym, work on myself, and meet new people at school. I had one person in mind who liked me in high school. That person, who often attended Jesus Camp, (what she called it) shall remain nameless. At first, I did not want to pursue it. I could not text her. We wanted to hang out when she came back from the camp.

> Bone marrow aspiration and bone marrow biopsy are procedures to collect and examine bone marrow — the spongy tissue inside some of your larger bones. Bone marrow aspiration can be performed alone, but it's usually combined with a bone marrow biopsy. Together, these procedures may be called a bone marrow exam.
> -The Mayo Clinic-

Since I have overcome cancer, I felt like I could overcome anything. My possibilities were endless. So, I finally got the courage and planned to ask her out after my 100th day of my bone marrow transplant. She was still the same: shy, cute, and funny. I thought she liked me, but I was terrible at reading women.

By the end of the summer, it felt amazing to take a full shower. I missed it. The doctor's appointments continued. I had three doctor's appointments in one week: one for my regular checkup, a second for my ultrasound, and a third because I was dehydrated from my first appointment. During the ultrasound check-up, the doctors found a high potential for a blood clot where my Trifusion Port was. So, good thing they were able to remove it. My doctor decided I did not need to take blood thinners. I did not have to redo the Lumbar Puncture Procedure. After Day 100, I could clean my house, walk the dogs, go on vacation and the beach.

On Lauren's birthday, the group planned a surprise at Fun Depot. The details, however, were vague. I received a text at 11:30 pm asking where I was. I was mad that no one told me what time to be there. I had no car and no money. I decided to stay home and catch up with them later when they would cut the cake. I asked for the cake cutting time, but I received no response for four hours! By the time I got an answer, they were already there. At that point, I said forget it! I was annoyed and hurt. I did not even tell Lauren Happy Birthday. I did not feel like anyone cared.

We also celebrated Mikey's birthday. We tried hitting the 21 and older clubs because some guy was handing out free tickets, but they turned us away. We even tried a strip club but didn't get in there either. We spent our night smoking hookah. I barely smoked because it wasn't healthy for me.

On Sunday, I visited my uncle's church and brought Matthew and Mikey along as they held a basketball tournament after the service. There were four teams, one referee and a prize for the winning team. We won one and lost another. Mikey and I did not play too much, which we were ok with. But Matthew and my cousin Mardoshe had lots of playtimes and did very well. It was a lot of fun hanging out with my cousin Mardoshe, as I don't get to see him often.

I asked my doctor what to say to my friends when they asked how I was doing physically. He replied, "Tell them it's too soon to call." I was hoping for him to say you are cured or don't have cancer anymore. He also said my Bone Marrow Biopsy looked very good, and he was sure the PET Scan would be good. My doctor discontinued two of my medications. I am not consuming as many pills each day. He increased my

Tacrolimus because my levels were off. Since my 100th day was approaching, he wanted another lung test in Deerfield Beach and a Pet Scan in Miami.

My diet had improved. Brandon referred us to this Ramen restaurant called "Cha-Cha" that serves the best food. Jordan and I went there, and the food was great, so we decided to make the place a regular. During one of our visits there, Jordan and I whispered to each other our waitress was low-key cute. I told him to ask for her number. He did not want to, so I decided to help him out. I put his phone number on my receipt before we left. It was hilarious. He got so mad. The girl never hit Jordan up. She probably thought we were some thirsty guys. I gained 3 pounds the first week I could eat out. My parents noticed I looked more muscular and were happy. My dad planned to get me started in soccer again, and I thought about playing for the Recreation Center.

Around that time, I saw an interesting movie called Sausage Party and saw Drake in concert with friends. It was a fantastic experience. During the movie outing, I saw my dawg, Patrick. He hasn't tied up with summer camp anymore, so I saw more of him. I went out for ice cream with the girl I was talking to. She is so pretty and sweet. Honestly, I do not even know if I have a chance with her. She might be out of my league. I hung out at Iyana's house as her parents were gone for the weekend. We just hung out and acted like teenagers. It was fun being myself and all silly with them. It has been way too long. Things were starting to feel normal again. I loved it!

Two bad things happened that summer. Luis moved to Virginia with his family. And my sister Carmie got into a bad car accident with my car. It was not her fault, though. The light turned green. Car one suddenly hit the brakes, causing car two to swerve out of the way. Car three (my car) hit car one. The two cars got minor damage. But my car airbags deployed, so it was totaled. The ironic thing is that Carmie returned from getting the title to her new car. Carmie was alright; she had some minor head damage. The muscle relaxers helped her out, though. I was so upset. I listened to John Mayer's Gravity the whole night. I was so down and needed someone to talk to. I texted this girl I was interested in, but she didn't answer, so I fell asleep to John Mayer. I woke up an hour later with a text saying she was sleeping. I told her I needed someone to talk to because the day was crappy. She said sure, and we spoke for a good hour. It is funny how things work out, though. I lost something important to me that day (my car), and God provided me with something else or, better said... someone else. I learned a lot about her, too, and her voice sounded so comforting on the phone. It was nice. Everything happens for a reason! That was my slogan. It helped me get through the toughest of times.

Besides fighting cancer, asking Elizabeth Marie to my second prom was the hardest thing I have ever done. I explained to her I had hoped to go with Lauren to my senior prom but had to decline because I was scheduled to be in the hospital for another chemo cycle. I asked her if she was going with anyone. She said no and laughed because she thought it was funny that I thought she had already found a date. How couldn't she find a date, though? I told her she is intelligent, hilarious, beautiful, ambitious, and has deep faith. All the guys at her school are completely blind. But even if she goes alone, she'll have fun.

She agreed to go with me, and I was excited and ready to have a nice night. That was until she told me she had to work because her boss was getting married. I wondered if that was a cover story because she did not want to go to my second prom with me, after all. Her friend ended up telling me she did not like me, and her mom did not want her to go with me because I'm black. Emotionally, I was destroyed.

Then I dreamed about her. I was in a crowded cafeteria in a college. I started to leave, but I heard someone call my name. It was Elizabeth Marie. I was surprised and happy to see her after such a long time. By her smile, I could tell she was so glad to see me as well. We hugged each other. Then I started to cry, which didn't make any sense. We left together, and by the door, we saw her friends. I noticed one of them was acting weird and hinting that we were together. I remember sitting in the passenger seat of Elizabeth Marie's jeep. The sunroof was up. She played music. It was perfect.

I woke up in the middle of the night, completely confused. I went on her Instagram because I couldn't seem to get her off my mind, and I wanted to know why I had dreamt about her. She looked twice as better as the last time I saw her. I had no idea she had a Jeep until I saw it on her Instagram page that night. I found it coincidental and exciting that I was with her in the same jeep in the dream. I thought about her that night; I did not care; I was sick.

I asked Luis if anything like this had happened to him when he was in treatment. He told me it was all me. It has nothing to do with the chemo and that he has been there before. He told me that I was a blessing. We ended up agreeing I should pray on it. I also told Patrick about the dream, who said that maybe the dream meant my family and friends love me or perhaps I like her. I told him I never stopped liking her. I felt pretty shitty after she pulled the plug on our prom date. He told me I could do way better. I shared I cannot even do better than my ex because I have no confidence. He agreed with Luis and suggested that I should go after Elizabeth Marie. I prayed my heart out that night.

Visiting My Alma Matter: Palm Beach Central High

I wanted to see Elizabeth Marie and my friends who were still in high school. So, Mikey, Patrick, and I went to Palm Beach Central High. I threw on my freshest set of clothes, which did not fit well, but I did not care. As I got to the front office with Mikey, I realized so much had changed since my graduation two years earlier. The rules were stricter, and the teachers were meaner. Even sign-in to enter the school ground was different.

Lauren walked in while I waited for Mikey to complete the sign-in sheet. We hugged, and she complimented me on my look. I said thanks and complimented her on her outfit as she always dressed well. Patrick walked in, and the same went down with him and Lauren. We made it to the door of our former Chorus class. Patrick and I argued about who should go in first while Mikey and Lauren laughed at us for being idiots. eventually won, and he went in last. As I walked in, everyone gasped and shrieked. We tried to walk in discreetly and slowly, but everyone saw us. Mr. Houchins, our Chorus teacher, was not too happy about disturbing his class. It felt like the old days.

> When it comes to cancer, many people believe that your life is completely over and you cannot live at all, but that isn't true.

Lauren went back on the choir stands, and Mikey, Patrick, and I sat to the side of class. My former classmates kept turning around and waving at me. Quietly, I ate my donut, trying not to disrupt the class. I played games on my phone as Mikey and Patrick quietly laughed. I raised my head occasionally to look for Elizabeth Marie.

As the bell rang, the students ran off the stands to grab their favorite seats at the cafeteria or get in line for their favorite food while my friends raced to see me. It felt like I had not seen them in years. They grew up and seemed more mature. I hoped life would be kind to them and that none of them would go through what I was going through.

During the lunch period, I joined Mikey as we visited some of our former teachers. We looked around, but some were on lunch duty, some had different classes, and some did not work there anymore. It was sad how much things had changed. Lunch was about to end, and I still hadn't seen Elizabeth Marie. I thought she skipped chorus class and went home early. I was a bit upset because I looked forward to seeing her.

Lauren wanted me to stay and hang out with everyone after class, but I wasn't feeling it. I also promised Mikey I'd drive him to see his girlfriend, so we left soon after watching Traditions Rehearsal--the chorus class I was part of. They sounded pretty good, but their style wasn't as lit as our class was.

Later that day, I spoke with Elizabeth Marie and learned that she was not in chorus anymore. She was doing well but stressed and tired of school. She was a graduating senior with two jobs. She seemed surprised at my promise to attend her graduation.

I filled her in and explained how I had to get a Bone Marrow Transplant. She shared how busy she was with her two jobs and dual enrollment at Palm Beach State College. I was anxious to see her. I asked if she wanted to have lunch the following Sunday after attending Christ Fellowship. She said yes but invited a friend along too. So, I invited Mikey to level the playing field. Her friend had a little too good of a Saturday night and did not wake up Sunday morning. Then after church, she bailed because she had last minute plans with her family. I died inside and cried to my boy Mikey.

Later, I went to the beach with Gabby, Mikey, Patrick, and Liz. I asked Elizabeth Marie, but she was working and could not make it. I did not get in the water, and everyone turned up, but I still had fun. The feeling of being out there, feeling the sand, smelling the sea and tasting the salty sea water made me feel new again.

I am still trying to crack the dream I had about Elizabeth Marie. I felt pretty good after having a great day at the beach, so I texted her as I often do to see how her day was. I also asked her if she was busy the next night. She said she was free. I did a little dance and then asked if she wanted to go to the movies. She said yes, and I did another dance.

The next day, I went to the mall with Mikey to see if I

could get my phone fixed. Before we left, I checked to see if Elizabeth Marie was working because, in my head, it felt like I hadn't seen her in years. I saw her. Even at work, the girl looked stunning. We hugged, and I died inside. Right there and then is when I started liking her again. She told her manager about me and how I was the friend she had mentioned a few months back. She remarked that I looked different and had lost a lot of weight. I told her I had heard that a lot lately. I did not stay too long because I did not want to get her in trouble with her manager. I also saw my homegirl Lauren who worked right across from Elizabeth Marie. I missed working and having responsibilities like them. I could not wait to get back to that life.

I dropped Mikey off at his house went home to get ready for the movie. I put on my best outfit as I was trying to impress, but it was hard with hair loss, atrophied muscles, and lack of confidence. But I had high hopes for the night.

I drove to City Place to meet Elizabeth Marie. I met up with Elizabeth Marie and her little sister, whom I was not expecting, but I played it cool. It took us so long to park that we ended up missing our movie. So, we went for ice cream. Her little sister went crazy because the ice cream parlor was filled with sweets and candies. I would've too, but I was trying to keep it cool.

While we waited in line, we talked. She said, "there's so much candy in this place that you could go diabetic." I responded, "too late!" and her jaw dropped open in shock. I laughed at that. I explained the whole situation about being diabetic, what happened to me in Boston, and why I looked so thin. She repeatedly mentioned how different I looked; the constant reminder hurt me. I felt she meant different in a negative way. But I played it cool as I knew I would get better. I also felt she did not mean to offend me. After I revealed what happened to me in Boston, she felt compelled to share something about herself.

She told me that she had been going to the doctor

lately because she may have a cancerous cyst in her ovaries. I wanted to die right then and there. I don't even remember what I told her afterward.

We walked around City Place. I dropped ice cream on myself and joked around. I shared how I couldn't fight off a dude to save them because I was weak. Also, they could beat me up and take my money. It was funny. But throughout the evening, I could not get what Elizabeth Marie revealed about her health out of my mind.

We sat by the docks and talked about our future. She planned to major in International Business, and I planned to major in Business Administration. She wants to get out of the country. I did too, but it wasn't the right time for me. We shared that we wished to have kids during this conversation, which was weird. Over dinner, we spoke about prom and college. Then we took the trolley back to where she parked.

Elizabeth Marie offered to drop me off at my car, so I would not walk this late by myself. We got in her car, the Jeep, precisely as I saw in my dream and blasted Uber after she told me she loves country music. I expected Eric Paisley.

When we got to my car, we said our goodbyes. I drove home, holding back tears from what she told me about her health. Picture me listening to John Legend with tears running through my cheek as I drive. It was terrible. I was not crying over a girl. I was crying because of what could happen to her. Since I could not get it out of my mind, I texted her to let her know it was eating me up. She told me not to worry about it and pray for her as the doctor needed to run a few critical tests before finding out if it was cancerous. I hoped that it was not.

My second prom and battle with self-image

I went to prom for the second time by myself after being admitted again to receive another round of chemo in the Jackson Memorial Hospital in Miami. This time, I brought my

Xbox. Time there flew by; I played COD with Mikey and stayed up late every night on my laptop.

The first week was easy. The Lumbar Puncture procedure went well, but I had the worst headache when I got back to my hospital room. I could not sit or stand up. I went home with this headache, and it did not go away for another week. I questioned my doctors about it. They said it was a side effect of the Lumbar Puncture Procedure because spinal fluid leaked out during the procedure, causing an imbalance in fluids, which caused the pain.

Although I was in the hospital with pain, I waited for Elizabeth Marie to text me her lab results. After my stay in the hospital, I went to Iyana's play with flowers to support her. It felt good to do stuff like that. I felt normal. The show was pretty good. I sat with a few of her friends, and it was a great night. It was an excellent way to come back home.

Because I did not know in advance whether I would make it to my second prom, I did not have a date. Lauren asked me to go with her, but I told her to find another date because I wasn't 100% sure I was going. So, she went with Vinny who is a good friend. Matthew said I should have asked Elizabeth Marie, but that ship had sailed even if I wanted to.

Prom weekend, I invited Lauren to my house to catch up. It was nice seeing her again. When she came over, "The Walking Dead" season finale was on, which she did not want to miss. Gabe invited us over to his house to watch it. Gabe, Alex, Albert, and a few of their friends went there; it was nice to see them.

Everyone was enjoying the show, and I looked uninterested. Lauren asked, "Are you ok?" I responded, "Yes, but I am in a ton of pain with this headache." Then, she started to massage my head, which felt amazing but wasn't doing anything for my headache. I rested my arm and head on the armchair, not paying attention to the TV. Lauren saw my pain and asked Gabe if I could lie down on his bed. He agreed. I passed out for about an hour and woke up in time to see the show's ending.

I dropped Lauren off at home, and she demanded I call her once I got home so she would not worry. I called her once I got home, and we spoke a little. We talked about Prom, and she suggested a blue tux, white shirt, and white pants. I was not feeling the white pants. I told her that I planned on spending a lot of money on my second prom and getting my outfit at H&M.

The following day, I brought my second prom outfit and saved a significant amount of money on this H&M sale. I saw Elizabeth Marie at the mall Kiosk when I got my prom outfit. She spoke with my friends, but not me. I was confused. I confronted her in the parking lot and asked why she did not respond to my text earlier. She said she was busy. She had a ton of stuff to do and a lot on her mind. The next day I texted her, and I got no response. I did not know what I did for her to treat me the way she did, but there was nothing I could do about it.

When Prom Day came, I was excited. The boys and I posed in front of my car and took great pictures. Then I stopped at Skyler's, who told me that I needed to pick up a gift from Elizabeth's girlfriend. It was a note and a bad hair day beanie. I appreciated her and the present; she is a fantastic friend. Then I drove to Iyana's house and saw a group of friends. WE ALL LOOKED HOT!!! We took a few pictures and then went to the Polo fields for more. We got an Uber ride to prom.

We jammed out to music and got hype for the fun night ahead of us. We went through the line for our wristbands. I saw some of my favorite teachers and former classmates from high school that night.

They were thrilled to see me. Everyone was surprised. Someone even thought I had moved to Boston for good.

I got a drink. I walked around and saw many of my soccer friends. We caught up a little about travel and college. One friend planned to attend the University of Central Florida with another member of our old soccer team. He said, "We should all room together." I told him, "We'll see" because of my health. I greeted a lot of people and reconnected with old friends. We got some food and sat at our table. Gabe had a sash on because he was running for Prom King. While I was

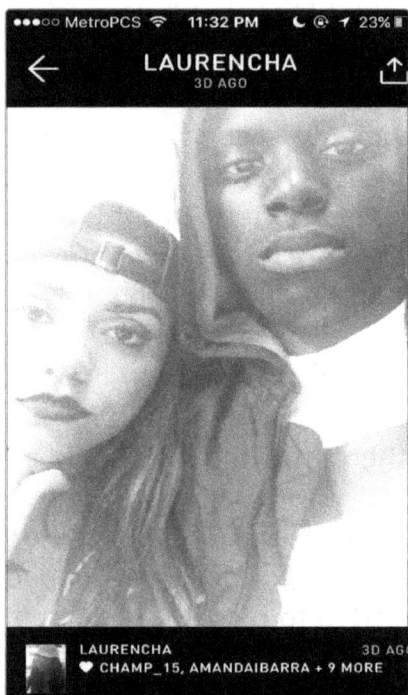

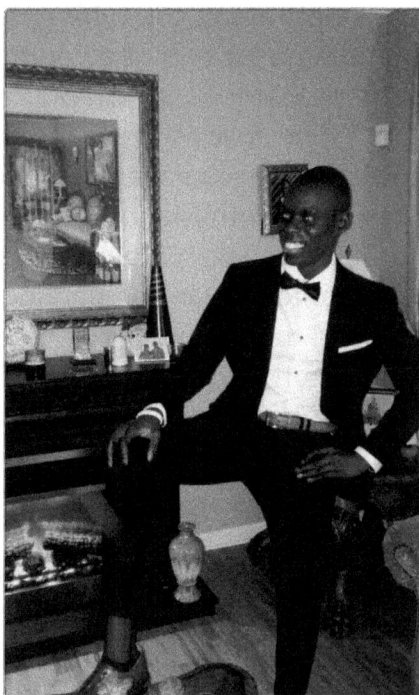

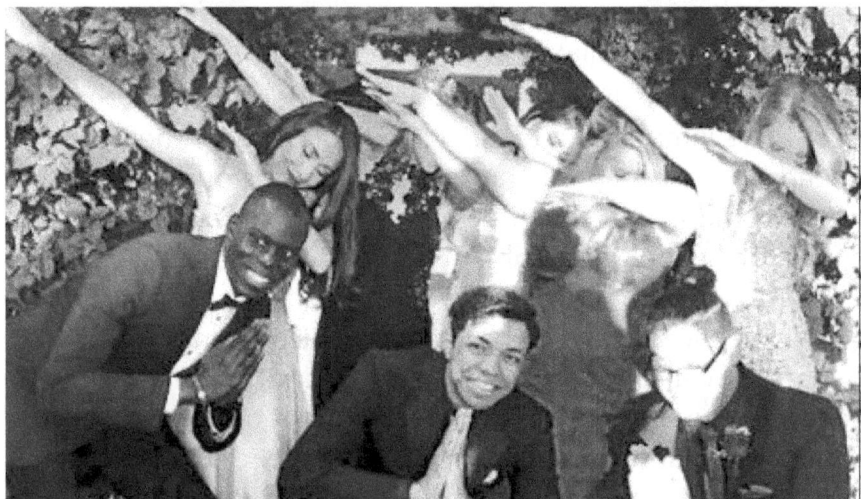

in Boston, Gabe met his girlfriend at a worship conference in Orlando. It was finally good to meet her; she was very nice.

I hit the dance floor and tried to dance as best as I could.Due to the loss of strength in my legs, I struggled, but I did a lot better than a lot of these guys who had no rhythm. Occasionally, I saw a big circle break out of nowhere and some girl throwing it back on another dude, in the craziest way possible; dudes hopping around to their favorite song and people dancing while recording everything on their phones. I was getting into it too. When "6 Foot 7" foot came on, I went in. I knew Lil Wayne's whole line. Everyone was lit for a good 30 minutes. Then the DJ played Bachata. I asked Lauren to dance. I did well until I tripped over myself, but I was having fun. Then, "One Dance" came on, and my friend Shela decided to dance with me. She said, "last year's prom was fun the whole night, and this year is boring." She was not wrong because everyone was throwing it back last year, not just a few girls. I am pretty sure I threw it back at one point. We even had a conga line!

I felt terrible because we barely danced. I am pretty sure I figured she stopped because I was too short. If I did not have chemo a week ago, I probably would have been able to touch the floor. The music stopped, and then they announced prom king and queen. It was Gabe and this pretty girl. It was not a shock that Gabe won, but everyone said Star won because of her looks. Gabe is such a clown that he did not even touch her when he was dancing because his girlfriend was there. I hit the dance floor and tried to dance as best as I could. After that, we all danced a little and took pictures at the photo booth.

Chapter Seven

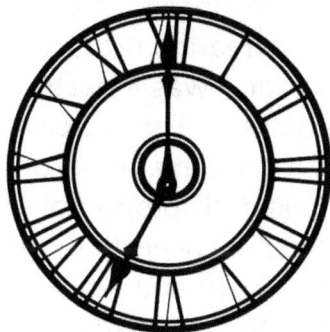

Graph Vs. Host Disease (GVHD)
Fall 2016

September flew by. I spent more than half of it in the hospital. A colonoscopy test showed that GVHD was at level 3 in my stomach and level 4 in my colon. The colonoscopy was probably the worst test I have ever had done. The preparation was the worst part. I could not eat anything solid for 24 hours. I had sugar-free popsicles and chicken broth. Since I was diabetic, I took steroids at home before being admitted. My body stopped absorbing food or medications. I was not eating, and I lost 20 pounds in two weeks. I had loose stools. *Crazy right?* The plan was to admit me only for a few days to take medications by IV (Intravenous Line) and discharge me when my stool formed. I planned on missing only about a day or two from school.

But the doctors did not discharge me as planned because of the loose stool. I ended up staying at the hospital for another 12 days. I missed so much school that I had to re-enroll for the next semester. I became depressed again. All my aspirations in life vanished. Once again, I stopped texting my friends and using social media. I tried to accept this without losing myself. I tried to focus on things I could control. Nephtalie stayed with me most of the time, so I bonded with her. JD, Jordan, and Matthew came by for a day.

After being in the hospital for 15 days, I gained all the weight. The steroid treatment that was helping fight the GVHD also made me eat. I was ingesting breakfast, snacks, one lunch, and two dinners. The steroids also did make me temporarily diabetic. It gave me a ton of pimples and made my face round. I looked disproportionate. I had to sleep in a chair because I experienced the worst pain in my legs whenever I tried to lay down and sleep. I couldn't walk at all. I cried. At first, the doctors gave me Morphine for the pain, then changed to hot patches. The hot patches helped at first, but they burned.

I was so ready to go, and I was looking forward to volunteer, with my friends and family, at a 5K run that was being hosted by POST. I texted Nadia to see if she wanted to volunteer with me, but I got no response. So, I deleted and blocked her number. I was done. Completely. I needed to move on. Last week, I told Skyler that I put others ahead of myself too much, to the point I end up hurting myself. I needed to start watching out for myself when it comes to situations like that. Well, you live, and you learn, right? I did not live ... I know. I have not been living lately, besides the Drake concert and my second Prom night. All I am doing is learning with no follow up. I plan to start living more when I get out.

> **I plan to start living more when I get out.**

Late falls and early winter months were much fun. We had a small gathering for my mom's birthday in October. Mikey graduated from broadcasting school. In early

September, Hurricane Hermine scared the whole state. I had another colonoscopy, and it showed no signs of GVHD. I saw my endocrinologist about my steroid-induced diabetes and a physical therapist to help with my workout. My goal was to get the water weight off and get my face to look normal.

On October 24, Lia slid into my DM on Snapchat. She attended my church a few years back. We started talking. At first, I helped her edit her first video vlog. I showed her my acceptance video for "3 little birds," which moved her to tears. We started hanging out with friends; we went to the beach and even did an escape room outing with Mikey and Jhamil. We got close. The down part is that she lives in Miami. She's in theatre school and works for a modeling company. I only saw her once a week on Saturdays when we were both free.

I went trick-or-treating on Halloween with Mikey and Jhamil. It was probably the last time we would do that because we were getting too old. November came around, and Trump became president. I was not the happiest about that because I was rooting for Hillary. Many people have mixed emotions about him. But I'll allow him to do his job. I can say this year, I got into politics and would love to pursue it someday. Recently, I have done some public speaking. At church, I spoke and told everyone about my journey, how I am not sick anymore, and thanked them for their prayers. I was losing a lot of the Prednisone weight, and physically, I felt good. The doctor cleared me to eat sushi and Subway at my own risk. He even cleared me to play soccer. All these things did not sit too well with my mom. But she must let things get back to normal. Next semester, I am starting school again with two online classes and one on-campus to make me feel normal. I recently trained with an old soccer coach who said he could get me back in a year. I know it will take a year because I can barely run one lap. He was the coach who recommended me to play for Haiti before I got sick.

I re-enrolled in classes and adjusted to college life

easier than I thought. But I had so much free time because I could only take a few classes. I tried to find ways to make money. I planned to push my music and get myself on the radio. Things were looking good until I started to experience symptoms of Graph Vs. Host Disease (GVHD). I was getting very itchy and had bumps everywhere. My doctor raised my Tacrolimus and put me on steroids, which made it better. A few weeks later, I started to see the side effects of the steroids; I noticed white bumps in the back of my throat because of being taken off anti-fungal medication. The doctor put me back on the medicine, and my throat cleared. However, my Tacrolimus levels were still off. I had terrible bowel movements. My mom gave me Imodium®, which helped a little. At this point, I have doctor's appointments twice a week, and my latest blood work shows that my sugar is elevated quite a bit. I checked my blood sugar and retook insulin. Also, I watched my intake, although I was not even eating one full meal a day. I do not know how things turned so wrong so quickly.

I was working out, eating well, and super happy not too long ago. Now I feel depressed half the time. I honestly could not help it. I had so many things weighing down on me. Lia isn't responding to my text. She promised to go out with me; I asked her about it, but no response. What the heck? That is rude. Sometimes I wondered if she even cared. Then I wondered if I should care. It seemed like a lost cause. I was not happy. I felt useless and unappreciated.

A Year Ago...

November 21, 2016, marked a year since I was officially diagnosed with Lymphoma. It was crazy how much I had gone through and was doing well. I am proud to say that I am CANCER FREE! Last year, I had to stop everything and head to Boston. It was terrible. I called everyone on my contact list and let them know I was leaving in one day. It was hard on everyone, seeing their faces at the airport at 4:00 am watching me go, uncertain whether I would return. Now I am doing better, and life has opened many doors. I have met a lot of people and experienced a lot. Looking back to the first day of getting to Boston, finding out I might not ever have kids and that I could die from all of this destroyed me, but it did not stop me from fighting for my life. God has blessed my life from being scared out of my mind on November 21, 2015, to being a hopeful, proud, brave, thankful young man. I'm happy that I'm alive, I'm glad to see my family every day, I'm so happy that many people love me, I'm so excited to be happy, and this is a blessing, a pure blessing. I AM NOT IN BOSTON. I AM NOT DEAD; I AM HOME, ALIVE, AND BREATHING on November 30th, 2016.

Thanksgiving was fun. I enjoyed it. I saw all my family, and I am glad to know that they are all doing well. I ate a lot of food and had so many leftovers. Things at home are still a little shaky. I hope everything goes well for my family. Sometimes I feel like we love each other but do not like each other very much.

> *God has blessed my life from being scared out of my mind on November 21, 2015, to being a hopeful, proud, brave, thankful young man.*

Things with Lia were back on track; we hung out, planned trips together, video chat till late in the night, and phoned each other all the time. We were both into what we had. A year ago, my mom told me she wished me to be in the position I am now: happy, going to school, a job, and a girlfriend. I am blessed, and I am so glad.

Luis came down with his family from Virginia for Thanksgiving. He never went back up with them. One night, I got a text from him letting me know he needed a place to crash. He did not sound very well. When he slept over, he told me about what had happened. If I realized one thing, he was constantly talking to God. I am glad that he knows that

God is always there for him and taking care of him. That man is a trooper. I encouraged him and shared that God would provide if he followed him; he will take you where you need to go. I truly love God. He ended up with two jobs and got a permanent place to stay.

I love this time of year. Last year, even though it was not the best, I still enjoyed it with my mom. We watched holiday movies in the hospital. It was funny. Being born and raised in Haiti, she did not know who or what Charlie Brown was. This year is coming together well. I got everyone's gifts, and I enjoy Lia being here around my family. I am hanging with my friends a little more. I am still on Prednisone, but I control my sugar well.

Grandma is here.

I am glad she's here; it's always lovely to see her. I wanted her to meet Lia before she goes back to Haiti after the holidays. Everything feels just right. I am happy. Everyone is supposed to slide to the crib around 2:00 p.m. to open gifts; we will be having eggnog, build a gingerbread house, and bake cookies while listening to Christmas music. And later, we will watch an old Christmas movie. Then after that, we're all going to tonight's service at church. God has allowed me to get better and see another year. I'm thankful happy, and I feel blessed!

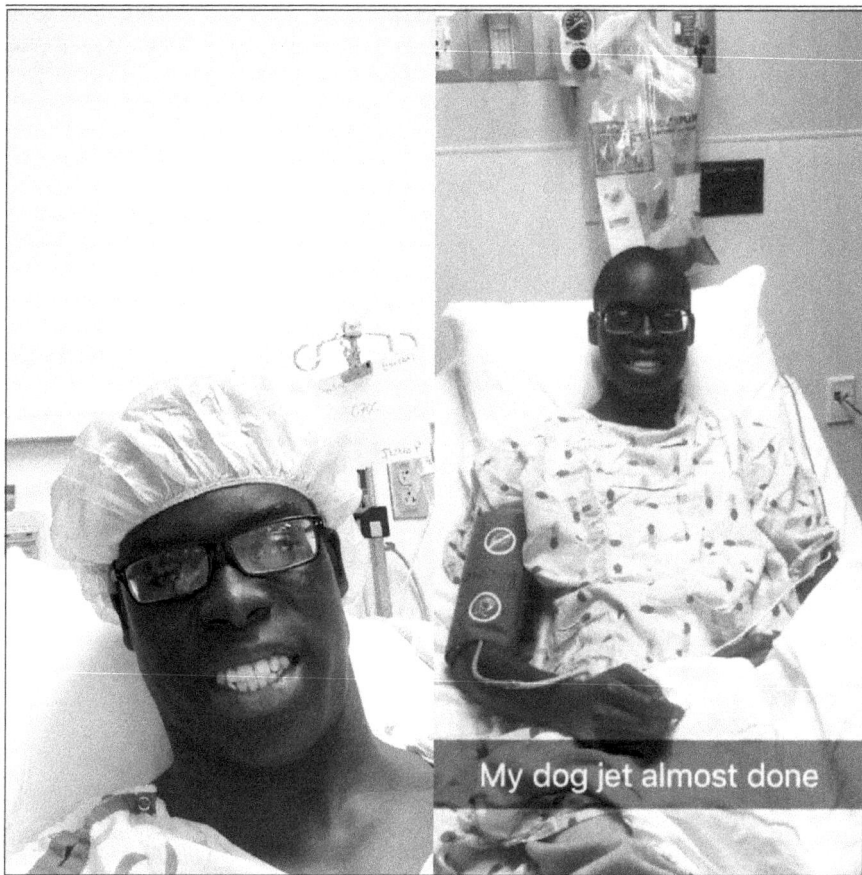

My dog jet almost done

Chapter Eight

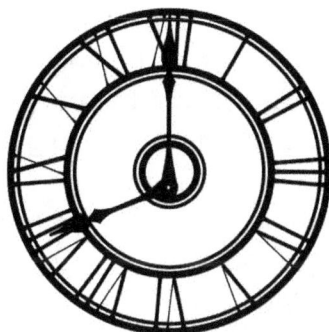

My Reality
January 2017

Since 2017 started, there have been plenty of ups and downs. Everything looked great spiritually, financially, and physically. Matthew started working at Delivery Dudes. Lia, Patrick, Mikey, Jordan, and I finally went to Disney, and I enjoyed myself after many dilemmas. There was a small argument between Lia and me about insulin, but neither of us was into arguing about something so stupid. Then, I had a stressful week at work with complicated orders and dealing with difficult co-workers.

I celebrated my first birthday again; I was under the impression that I would have another big surprise party, but it did not happen. Instead, a fun family dinner outing occurred the night before my cousin's concert. Nephtalie got a job and was working 24/7. I was upset about that.

Every Saturday, I tutored math to a 4th grader with A.D.H.D. I also started a four-day tax course. If you can pay attention in the boring class, the work is simple. If you take your time and study, it's something anyone can do. So, I thought, until I went to take the exam. I exploded because there was so much going on with my medicine, health insurance, the class, and Lia. So, I turned off my phone and disappeared. I drove around Palm Beach went back to my roots, where I was diagnosed, my old daycare, house, and even the park. I got some food and a soccer ball. I planned to shoot around to clear my mind and reminisce, but the park was closed. I threw the ball over the fence and attempted to get over it, but I could not because I was too weak. So here I was on one side of the fence and the soccer ball on the other. It was sad. In my mind, this was a sign that I would never get back to soccer. That evening, I hung out with Lia at the South Florida fair, then dropped her home in Miami. I got home that night and cried to my mom. I found out my family and friends were looking for me. They almost called the police and hospitals. It was a crazy night. I was fighting with work because they fired me without an explanation. I thought I would be fine without a job. I had bigger things to worry about; family, school, music, and God, who has been taking care of me, and I trust him, so I'm good.

One early February morning, Lia texted me, and I started reminiscing about our relationship. We have a YouTube channel together; we are not arguing; we're enjoying each other and everyone around us. We are going out together, in constant contact over text, supporting each other, and it is excellent. When things get hectic, we speak and figure them out. When you love someone, you can get through the most challenging times.

I received positive feedback from the rhyme I released for Valentine's Day. I am getting along with my sisters more, and I love Carmie's relationship with my girlfriend. I have been eating well; protein shakes in the morning, protein shakes in the afternoon, and a healthy dinner. So, my sugar level was pretty good. I have been working out. I am regulated with 30 mg of Prednisone. I cannot wait until I am of these medications for good. It is honestly hard to look at myself right now. I feel terrible and have stretch marks everywhere. My weight was awful, but I am working out each morning. It takes time, but I feel like my self-esteem is damaged. Lia and I were being corny the other night, and we told bedtime stories. Her story told me that no matter how I look or how I am, she will always love me, just the way I am. Hearing that made me feel good, knowing that she would always be here no matter what.

My endocrinologist was impressed with my blood sugar level. I am off Tacrolimus, so I can go to the lake and wake up late if I want to. It feels great to say that! Lia posted a "How We Met" video on YouTube. She put a lot of hard work and effort into it. I am glad that she was still working on our projects even though I was busy. I appreciate all the hard work she does. That is Bae! Earlier, Jordan asked me where I was and how I was doing. It has been a while since we have chilled, so we planned to hang out soon. I lay in bed cool, calm, and collected, and it has been a while since I felt this way.

I planned to do a photoshoot in the morning with my girlfriend. I was upset that my tutoring appointment was canceled since I needed the money. I went to the pool for the first time over a year, and it was fun. Lia got her nails done as I waited for what seemed like forever. Afterward, I tried to prank Lia for our YouTube page with flour in her hair Dryer, baby oil in the shampoo bottle, and then icy hot in a toothpaste bottle. None of it worked. We volunteered with my sister at a Pink Stripes breast cancer fundraising event. I planned to take Lia out to dinner and a movie, but she preferred to stay at the Breast Cancer Awareness event since they were also hosting a fashion show as she is all into that. Lia plans to move back to her family home in West Palm Beach so it can be better for us as a couple. Occasionally, as with every relationship, Lia and I argue. But we try our best to fix things.

My body is feeling pretty good. I am glad the doctors decreased the Prednisone dosage, and my blood sugar is more regulated; my weight is also going down. I continue with my doctor's appointments, focus on school, and run errands with my parents. I am figuring out my future; there is not much weighing on my brain, so I enjoy working on myself and getting better physically. I have been reading my daily devotional more often. I learned that nothing could come into a man that can defile him, but what comes out of him is what defiles him.

In March of 2017, I started to experience another round of emotional ups and downs. But I can say that it's looking brighter. Because money was tight as the tutoring job ended and I was not optimistic, I stayed home almost the whole spring break, which helped me get a lot done. My uncle promised to find me another student to tutor. I

I was glad to see my friend Jhamil happy with his new girlfriend, who lives in Tallahassee. We are planning to see the new Power Rangers movie in the theatre. My friend Holger hooked Lia and me up with a video and pictures. That's what I call a great friend. We need more people like him around. I met Kelly, one of Lia's closest friends. We all hung out together at the pool, watched "Get Out" in the theatre (what a fantastic movie!), scouted for B.E.A.M. Squad at Aventura Mall (long story), and hung out at her place.

I have been making moves. I have been focusing on homework and recently found out I will be graduating next spring. I am very excited! Lia went to Pangea with her friends. She was a little too turn-up, but her friends were looking out for her. It was her last hurrah before going home. She looked amazing, but anything could have happened.

I picked her up from her place. Again, we argued about something dumb. I felt a certain way, so I took my feelings to Twitter. She did not like the arguing and the tweets. So, she broke up with me. Later, we made up after I apologized. She said she could not be without me and that she loved me. I agreed, and we planned to meet up to fix the situation. She is special to me, and I can't think straight when we argue. I love her so much. I met a lot of her friends at her welcome home party. I want to do something with just the two of us for her birthday. I have big plans, and I hope to get all of them done.

I have been healthy lately, and my doctors continue to be impressed and have decreased my Prednisone dosage.

I had one scary moment where I fainted for about 7 seconds. We believe one of the medicines I was taking caused it, which the doctor took me off very quickly. I am lucky Carmie was there to help me. I am happy and grateful for everyone in my life, good or bad. They have all helped shape me into who I am today, and I'm proud to be me.

My party for my second birthday is coming up in a few weeks. I cannot believe it is about to be April 26, 2017. I am almost done with school.

Unfortunately, Lia and I broke up after she promised that we would work things out. From what I understand, I edited some pictures that we took for her birthday after she told me not to. She also felt that she could not rely on me. Honestly, I think there is another reason. It is hard to move on, but I am looking. I do not want to do anything until I know that she is over me. She told me she still likes me physically and emotionally, but not mentally. She also told me it was overwhelming trying to make time to hang out with me. She did not even have time to hang out with her friends. She honestly does not know what she wants, and I'm not going to wait around for her to figure it out. She might find a boyfriend at work. All the guys there are into her. Who knows? Whatever happens, I will not be happy. Yes, I loved her, and I still do, but I think we shouldn't be together.

Lately, I have felt lonely and sad. I spend most of my time at home alone. Then when I go out, I am usually alone. No one hangs out with me. Even when I ask, I get no response.

I guess that is one thing about Lia. She was my best friend, and I would always be with her. I was never by myself when we were together. It wasn't hard for people to realize we had broken up because I was posting on my Snapchat alone, my Instagram picture was only of me, and my bio no longer had her info. When I try to figure out if she is still interested, she does not reply. If she does, it will be hours later, and it will be very brief and general. It seems that she only texts me if she needs something. Before my second birthday party, I dreamt of proposing to Lia with a promise ring at my party. I do not know if I was willing to go through with it. I feel like she is talking to someone right now. A few days after my party, she texted me asking for the start time. She acted like she did not know it was a few days ago, even though I posted online. I told her I got a job, and I also recommended her. It pays well, so I know it would help her out. I still love her a lot, but I do not think she's interested in getting back with me.

Matthew moved away. It is sad. I miss that annoying little child. I feel like I raised him. It will suck being without him, but that's life.

I gave a speech at my college (Palm Beach State). The response was very positive. The audience shared how my story touched and motivated them. That is all I ever want to hear from people. That means I am doing God's work.

Lately, I've been getting headaches, my back has been sore, and everything I eat gives me stomach aches. I hope it doesn't mean anything as I don't need another stay in the hospital. I got a job at Vector, and I think it will provide me with a promising future.

My fight with Graph Vs. Host Disease (GVHD)
March 2017- March 2018

I was readmitted to the hospital again because of food poisoning from Spaghetti that made my family and me very sick. The food poisoning increased my risk for GVHD.

I started to have gas and diarrhea all day. They did two Enemas and started to prepare me for a 10 am colonoscopy. There were complications with the scheduling, so it was rescheduled for later. I was not happy about prepping for no reason. I was hungry and had not eaten in 48 hours. My lunch and my breakfast were staring at me, but I couldn't eat them. If it weren't done, I would have to wait a month.

As part of the first treatment step for diarrhea, I take Prednisone. I was happy that I got off this medication. But now, I was back on it at a high dosage (80mg per day). They finally took me late in the afternoon. They brought me downstairs to the prep room and then back upstairs. By this time, I was distraught because I was starving. I prayed the colonoscopy was negative so I could go to a party, book my hotel for the Disney vacation, have a good weekend, start work, make money again, do well, and put this all behind me because this was all terrible.

When things start looking up, they always seem to take a turn for the worse. I was honestly sick and tired. My friends are on break from school; it seems like every time I am admitted, my friends are on vacation, makes no sense. I felt life loves to walk all over me sometimes. But God is good, and I must stay strong always... always... always....

As I am sure you can imagine, so much has happened. I started feeling down mentally and physically ... I wonder why? My health suffered, and I went to the clinic from passing out. My liver levels were terrible, and I got admitted to the hospital again. No surprise. I spent 22 days there, lost and confused. I met a good amount of new people. I did a few videos. I got my surgery recorded and was a star for a day. I was on a clear diet for five days. I could not eat, it was the worst, but it was not new. I had gone through many nights of tears, and I had to fight off taking pain medications. I hope to get out soon.

I was put on a new treatment. Whew! I must be in Miami three times a week for a Photopheresis test (it takes time to work.) Today I have done my thirteenth test, my left eye is super dry, and it is hard to open. I am diabetic again, and I cannot be in the sun because of the treatment. I cannot go to the pool because of the Trifusion I have in my chest, but my face looks better. I cut my hair. Hopefully, I can get it grown back with curls because my hair texture is different now.

I'm single, it's super official, and I'm not looking around, but hey, who knows? I have been keeping in touch with my family. We got back from a Disney trip, we even took the dogs, and I enjoyed myself. I'm mentally more stable and happier. I know there is a lot of evil but:

I am alive!
I can say I beat cancer.
No. My family beat cancer.
All of this is through the grace of God.
God has blessed my life from being scared out of my
mind from November, to now a hopeful, proud, brave, and
thankful young man.
My journey has God written all over it.
It hurts if I compare myself to my closest friends
and their accomplishments.
Don't get me wrong; I'm happy for them.
Even though there are times I feel I've done nothing
with my life, in comparison.
I've accomplished so much,
and this journal will not end here.
The same fire that got me through this still burns.

I hope you enjoyed it.
Until later.

Glory Be to God!
Jethro R. Pierre

Chapter Nine

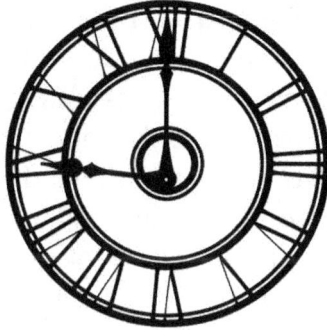

Jethro's Last Testaments

I am glad I decided to write down and share my journey. I feel no shame towards any of the content I have shared. My privacy is out there. I want you to connect and feel how this whole process truly felt. I believe it was the wisest decision I have ever made in my life! As for all my family and friends who have been a part of this arduous journey: I love you all, and I appreciate you being okay with all of this. So many people have contributed to making this journey unique, memorable, and authentic. I have changed in so many way. My outlook on life, my appearance, and so much more. This is the beginning for me and many others. I know it. I can feel it. I had planned to end this story on my second birthday on April 26th, but it did not seem natural enough to me. I wanted to give everyone all of me, every moment, down to the last minute.

- **Mom and Dad:** I wish there were something I could give you. Everything I am including my worldly possession, is from you two. You guys gave me a life worth living twice. Because of you two, I am the man I am today. I thank you for that, and I could never repay you for that.

- **My sisters Nephtalie and Carmie:** You guys made my life enjoyable. From beating me up for fun to being there with me when I am at my lowest. I can say you two have been there for me. You are the only people that have seen me on my best and worst days. Carmie, despite what anyone says about you, I know you can pull through anything and make it far wherever your heart takes you. Naphtalie, stay focused and finish whatever you have started. I do not want me being gone to distract you. I expect some kids from you two. You've got years to make that happen, or I will haunt you. I am joking, or am I? I guess we will find out, ha-ha!!!

- **To all my aunts and uncles:** I have always appreciated the hard work you all put together into making this family. I know it was not easy at first, but you all fought hard to be where you are today. That always impressed me and inspired me to do better as an adult.

- **To my cousins that I feel distant from:** In the past, I preferred to stay home and hang out with my friends rather than visit my family. I wish I had prioritized both.

- **Yvelor, my cousin, but a brother:** How you created your family always inspired me to work hard so I can have a family like you have. A beautiful wife and son. God has blessed you in so many ways.

- **Jephte, my cousin, but a brother:** I don't remember a time when I wasn't looking up to you. It felt like I finally got a brother when you lived at my house. Like you, I wanted to play soccer and make music. You inspired me in many ways!

- **Hermeline, my cousin, but a sister:** Thank you for coming to see me in Boston. I enjoyed your presence. Stay the happy person you are. We need more people like you in this world.

- **Moline, my cousin, but a sister also:** I enjoyed growing up with you and your siblings. I miss and reminisce on the days of getting the remote for you when it was right in front of you.

- **Angela, my cousin, and another sister:** Life got hard for you just when things seemed to start falling into place. Just stay strong in faith and let everything fall into its proper place. Everything happens for a reason!

- **All cousins, but siblings:** We're the last generation, and I hope you guys go the distance.

To my close friends:

- **Matthew:** You have grown a lot (No pun intended). You are the closest person to a little brother. I contemplated roasting you in this. Do not get caught in the hype of life. Do things right. You can have my Drake CDs, and whatever you want in my closet.

- **Jordan, another brother:** We have been at it for a long time. Before I was friends with anyone else in Wellington, you were my first friend. I remember us shooting around on my messed-up basketball hoop. Those were the good old days. Jordan, you have everything set up for you in life. I know you might not see it sometimes, but you can thank your parents for that. Stay a good person, be yourself, and never doubt yourself.

- **Mikey, my older brother:** You are the only one I can get in an argument with, ruin my day, and make me feel terrible afterward. I care about you a lot. I know you can do something great in this world. You must believe in yourself. I promise you already have the tools; I see them. That is why at times, I get so aggravated at you. You have it, man. Keep faith in God, praise him, and let him do the rest. Things will slowly look better, I promise.

- **Skyler, another brother:** You have a great heart. Probably the best out of everyone. Keep your loved ones close, and do not get distracted. You have done a lot of maturing over the years as well. Figure out what you want in life, grab hold of it, and never let go.

- **Caillou, I'm joking, JD, another brother:** I'm glad that your family moved from Alabama to Florida. Many do not say it enough, but you're a good friend. It gets boring when you leave for the summer or whenever for Alabama. I always liked that you rep where you're from. Don't be afraid to show your feelings. Keeping it all in can make you go mad.

- **Ian, another brother:** I always saw a leader in you. I know you have what it takes to make reasonable changes in this world. Every time I see you, I still see the same kid I grew up with, even though we grew apart. You never changed. Stay focused.

- **Luis, my big brother:** You have helped me out so much on this road. You showed me many things about what I am going through. I want to say thank you. You did not have to do any of that, but you did because that is how great you are. You are not the type of person to leave someone in the dark. Never change, brother. You are a blessing. I know you have what it takes to make it far in life with music. Keep working on hard on your music.

- **Patrick:** We have a lot in common, from sports to chorus. It all happened so quickly. I could always tell you about any girl I have been crushing on, and you would always do the same. I am glad you finally found the one. At least one of us eventually did. Do not worry. I'll be at the wedding — in the back— in tears probably. You are a hard worker and a great friend. I wish the best for you in the future.

- **David, my brother:** Like Gabe and Alex, I always admired your faith in God. I probably would have been a worse person if it wasn't for you. I wish the best for you and Kenny, and I know you guys will be together even in the heavens.

- **Gabe, my brother:** I gave you the torch after I graduated, and you made the flames even bigger. You are a great friend, and I expect you to impact many lives in the future, as you did mine. I still remember that prayer the night before I left for Boston.

- **Alex, my brother:** You are a bright person. Always happy and in the moment. Keep that with you as you mature into adulthood because you will need that attitude in life.

- **Albert, my brother:** I have known you a short time, but it feels like I have known you forever. You have that effect on people. It was always fun hanging with you. Stay the same person and always show your true colors.

- **Gabby, one of my sisters:** You have helped me a lot through this tough road. I know life can get hard sometimes, but sometimes you must push through it and wait for better days to come. Keep in mind, there is always a rainbow on the horizon.

- **Elizabeth, my sister:** You always were blunt with me about any girl I liked and always was a good friend. You reminded me a lot of my older sister. Keep faith in God; he will take you far. He already has.

- **Iyana, my sister:** If it were not for you and your family, I would not have made it out of Boston at all. You guys honestly helped me get closer to God.

- **Lia, one of my exes:** Every time I see you, you have the brightest smile, one that lights up the whole room. I always loved that about you. You will be famous one of these days.

- **Tori, my sister:** You are the only friend who has seen and touched my port without freaking out. Be you and keep the right people around you.

- **Lauren:** You have supported me so much throughout this

journey; it is shameful how things have turned out. I always wanted something more than a friendship when the time was right, but I got distracted by the wrong ones, so who knows. Stay the strong individual you are, and do not let anyone or anything get in the way of your happiness. You are one-of-a-kind.

Epilogue by Hermeline Blanc
Jethro's cousin

March 2018 was a whirlwind. I never thought I'd spend a week in an Intensive Care Unit, then spend another week drafting a wake and funeral program, writing an obituary, a prayer, and creating a slideshow for my dear cousin Jethro Pierre's Celebration of Life events.

None of this was part of the plan. Indeed, we never know the day and the time when our lives will be turned upside down. My sister was supposed to spend the second week of March with me in New Jersey, where I live, and then we were going to travel to Florida together for a long weekend to celebrate my college friend's birthday. I was supposed to return to Jersey right after these fun celebrations.

There were no significant signs that this was the turn Jethro's health would take. On March 4, while crying in front of my building, my mom told my sister and me, "the doctors are asking for our family." At first, I thought, no! My mom is highly emotional and exaggerating. But my sister, who is a medical professional, looked at me and said, "Something is seriously wrong if they are asking for our family."

That same day, barely breathing with an oxygen mask, my cousin Jethro asked me, "Did you receive your birthday gift?" I said no and told my aunt to take the phone away and let him sleep. That was the last time I spoke with him. The hearty IHOP breakfast and the movie outing to "Black Panther," which my sister and I planned, no longer sounded appealing. My sister jumped on the computer and booked us flights to Florida.

By the time we got to the University of Miami Sylvester Comprehensive Cancer Center, Jethro had been intubated. We spent as much time with him as possible, both as a family and individually. We took turns singing, praying, crying, and laughing each night. As we waited, the doctors reaffirmed our worse fears every morning, but each night the ICU was booming with noise from our family and friends—hoping and praying for a miracle.

A week after my sister and I arrived, my cousin died right before our eyes at 8:14 a.m. on March 14. He passed from an irreversible inflammatory lung condition called bronchioles Obliterans, which affects the lung's tiniest airways. Simply put, he had respiratory lung failure because his lung wasn't getting enough oxygen.

We never expected him to die at such a young age and in such a manner. Up to his last breath, Jethro wanted to live. Watching him die was traumatic for every member of our family. I find comfort knowing my cousin impacted his world with only the 21 years he had.

We were born to give and receive love. Ultimately, love is what everyone remembers when we take our last breath. The time spent and the love shared are meaningful and indispensable. The time spent and the love shared are meaningful and dispensable. What we do in between are fillers. The time spent and the love shared are meaningful and dispensable. The lasting effect of our lives is wrapped up in love, which manifests through memories we leave behind. My cousin Jethro Pierre knew such wisdom of life and lived in such away. Jethro was tenacious about making a difference. His sense of humor made him a favorite. He helped his friends be more inclusive. He helped those around him realize life is not always about what we think is right. To my knowledge, he stopped one person from committing suicide.

In the ICU, medical professionals tend not to get personal with patients. But with Jethro, it was hard not to be. He was so unique and full of life even through his illness. The hospital staff loved him; they were supportive and even cried with us.

When he was alive, Jethro urged us to be open-minded. He is still doing that even after his death. That same college friend I was supposed to celebrate with the weekend Jethro passed dreamt that we were all around Jethro's bed crying and praying. Jethro sat up from his bed, took off his oxygen mask and looked at us with an attitude and overwhelming confidence (as he would in real life), and said, "Why are you guys crying? I am in heaven." He shakes his head and lays back to rest.

If that is not a confirmation that my cousin is no longer suffering, I do not know what is. We miss you daily, Jethro. Some days are worse than others, but by God's grace, we will be okay. Our family has a quiet strength, and we are closer than ever. Through Jethro's death, I learned that there is always a silver lining, and God has our backs no matter what this life brings.

My brother sang these words at Jethro's service, and they resonate with me every day, "They could never say that you didn't try. They could never say you didn't give your all...."

We cannot wait to see you in heaven, my dear cousin. Indeed, you tried with all your heart, might and strength. We'll love and remember you, always!

Digital Obituary

Obituary

Jethro Roosevelt Pierre of Wellington, Florida, Born January 23, 1997, went to be with the Lord on March 9, 2018, at 8:14 a.m. at the University of Miami Sylvester Comprehensive Cancer Center. Although Jethro won his battle over Acute Lymphoblastic Lymphoma, he died of an irreversible inflammatory lung condition called bronchioles obliterans, which affects the lung's tiniest airways.

Jethro fought a great fight; so, we can proclaim, "O death, where is your victory? O death, where is your sting?"

Jethro's love of people helped us see the silver lining during this difficult time. He urged all to look at different perspectives in life. When we, his family and friends, wouldn't get it, he would assert himself attempting to show us that everything was possible because he beat cancer.

Jethro's short 21 years of life were filled with impactful moments. He played travel soccer for Wellington Wave and varsity soccer at Palm Beach Central High. His stellar sportsmanship led him to play for the state of Florida Olympic Development Program. But as a family, we remembered his beginning days on the soccer field. We lovingly teased Jethro of his round eyeglasses, which he needed to do pretty much everything. Imagine a skinny little "Steve Urkle" running around the soccer field with a ball. Our family joked about how Jethro lacked the toughness to play sports because he refused to play rough. As one of the leading scorers, Jethro shared "moments of glories" with his teammates.

Jethro had an entrepreneurial spirit and wished to obtain a business degree. It was evident through various business ventures and his pursuit of knowledge. Jethro completed homework in the hospital room and got frustrated when we wanted him to focus on being healthier rather than his various projects.

Jethro was tenacious about making a difference. His sense of humor made him a favorite. He helped his friends be more inclusive. He helped those around him realize life is not always about what we think is right.

He started publishing his journal "But Seriously... Where did the time go?" in which he documented every step of his journey. As a family, we will ensure his book gets published. Jethro shared his journey at cancer support groups. He volunteered to feed the homeless, and when his disease progressed, he focused on developing his hidden gifts of music and writing. Jethro depicts his life through his songs entitled; I'll be free, Medication, Eat, Pray and Grind, among others. He wanted his story to comfort those battling any disease, especially cancer.

Jethro is survived by his parents, Roosevelt and Marie Pierre. His sisters Nephtalie and Carmie Pierre. His grandmother Anne Pierre; His aunts and uncles: Llyonel and Naomie Mercius, Gerard Meus and family; Manes Blanc, Jocelyne Mercius; Voltaire Estimable; Angeline Saintphard, Marie Pierre; Lucie Jean-Jacques, Julio and Grace Success, Michelle Corieorolant and family, Clarita Pierre; His cousins: Rushama, Madoshe, Misha, Jemima Mercius; Hermeline, Moline and Jephte Blanc; Yvelor, Jacques and Loudi Sully, Angela Saintphard, Sarah Paul; Isaac Jean-Jacques; Ruben, Getty Welger, and Wood Mercius; Manouscha, Kathy and Shapounah Mercius; Sadrack Mentor and Sabrina Bienaime; Philo and Wiggins success; Thompson and Rose Cesar; Regis and Uldah Success; Sadrack Mentor and Sabrina Bienaime and many more extended family as well as a multitude of friends and schoolmates.

A tribute gift can be made in the loving memory of Jethro Pierre instead of flowers to Pediatric Oncology Support Team, Inc. at http://postfl.org/donate/, which supports local children and their families who are faced with cancer in South Florida.

Safely Home

I am home in Heaven, dear ones.
Oh, so happy and so bright!
There is perfect joy and beauty.
In this everlasting light.

All the pain and grief are over,
Every restless tossing passed;
I am now at peace forever,
Safely home in Heaven at last.

Did you wonder I so calmly?
Trod the valley of the shade?
Oh! But Jesus' love illuminated.
Every dark and fearful glade.

And He came Himself to meet me.
In that way so hard to tread.
And with Jesus' arm to lean on,
Could I have one doubt or dread?

Then you must not grieve so sorely,
For I love you dearly still:
Try to look beyond earth's shadows,
Pray to trust our Father's Will.

There is work still waiting for you,
So, you must not idly stand;
Do it now, while life remained –
You shall rest in Jesus' land.

When that work is all completed,
He will gently call you Home.
Oh, the rapture of that meeting,
Oh, the joy to see you come!

-Unknown

In Memory of

Jethro R. Pierre

January 23, 1997 - March 9, 2018

Jethro's Life in Pictures

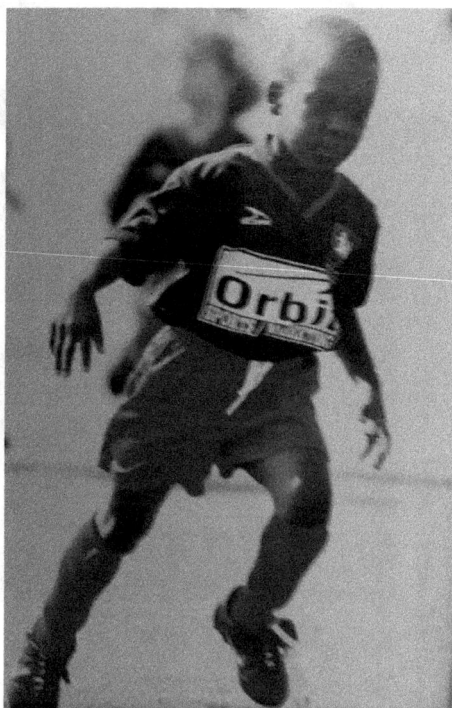

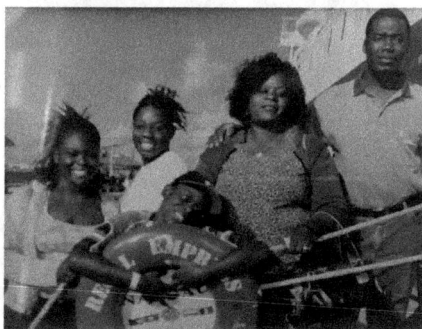

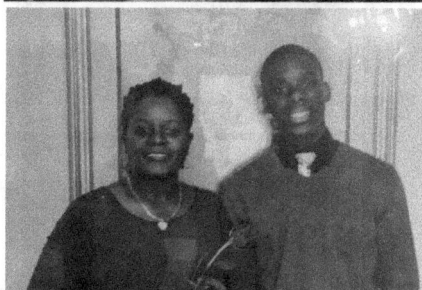

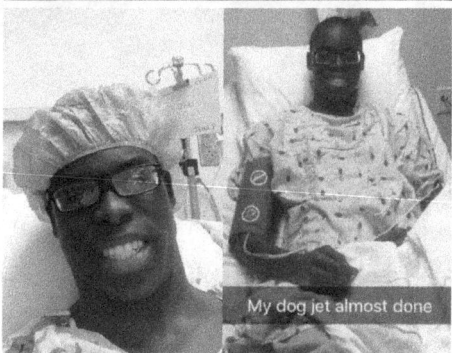

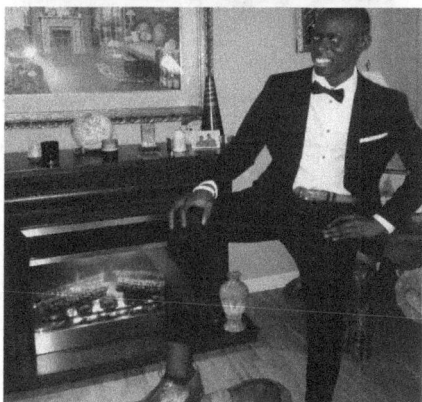

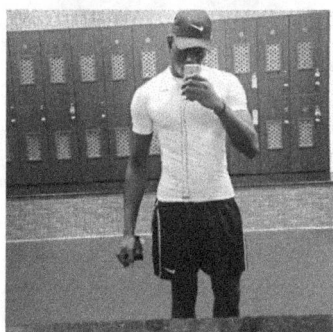

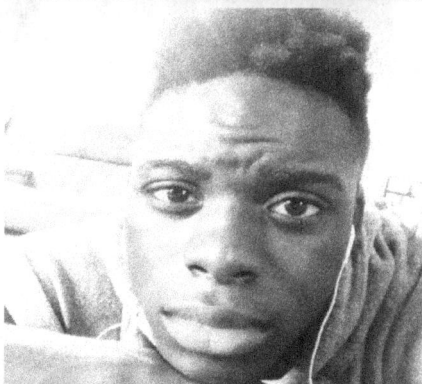

My dog jet almost done

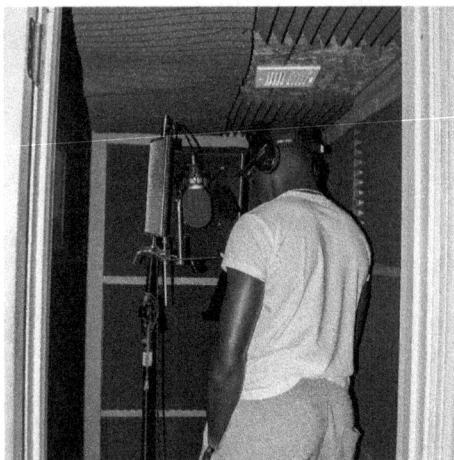
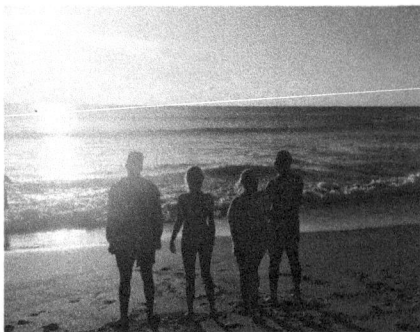
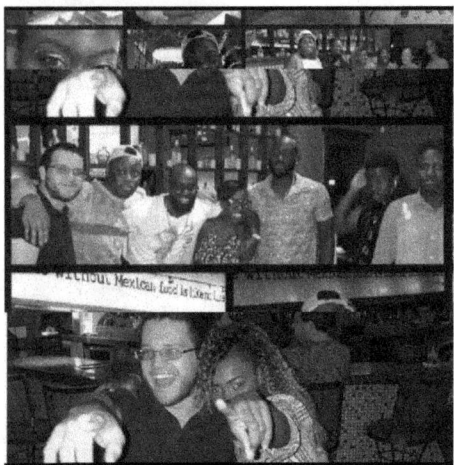
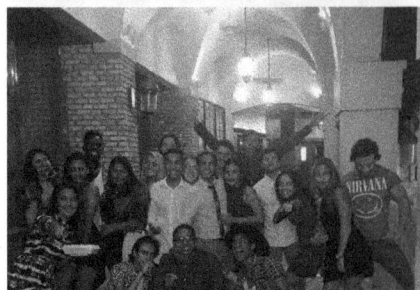
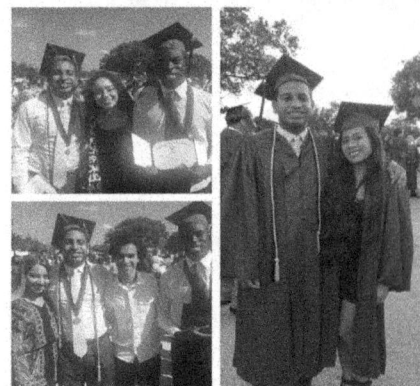
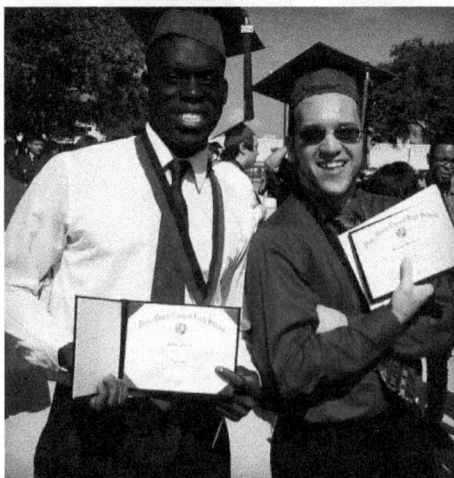
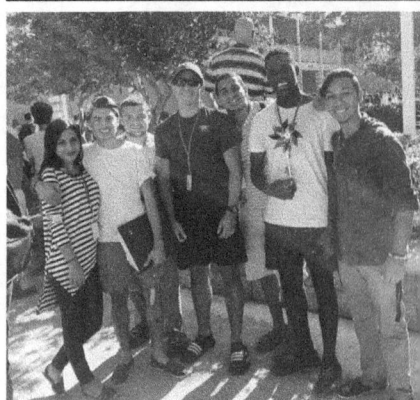

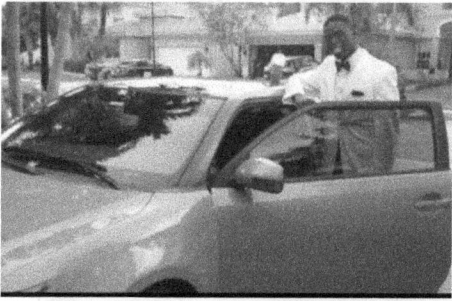

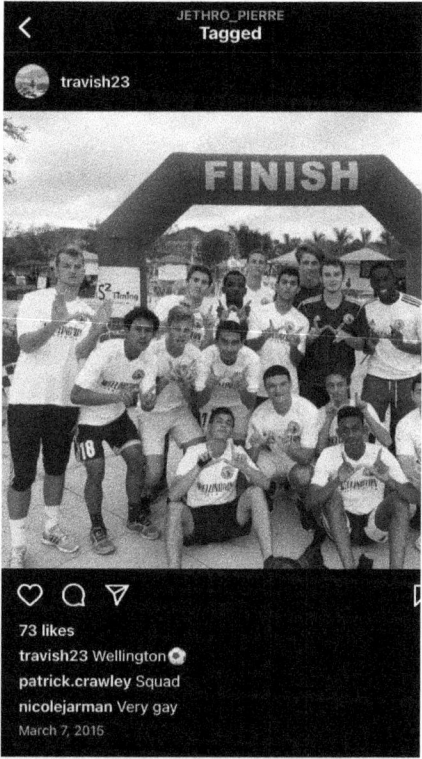

travish23

73 likes
travish23 Wellington ⚽
patrick.crawley Squad
nicolejarman Very gay
March 7, 2015

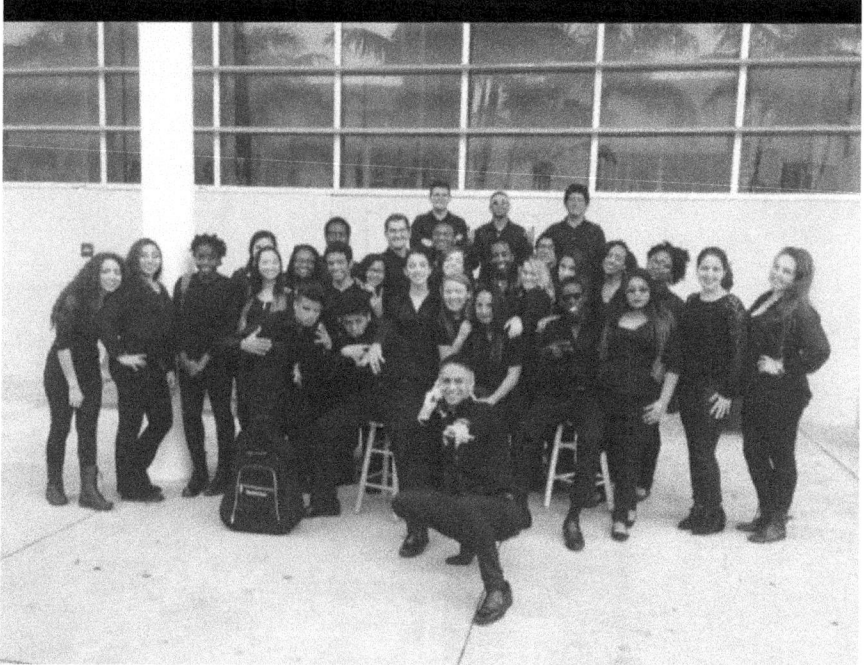

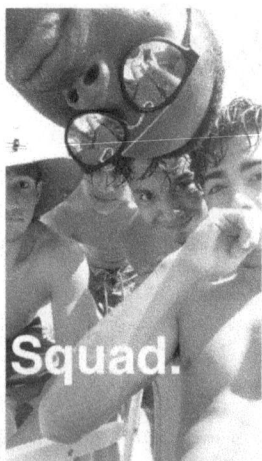

Squad.

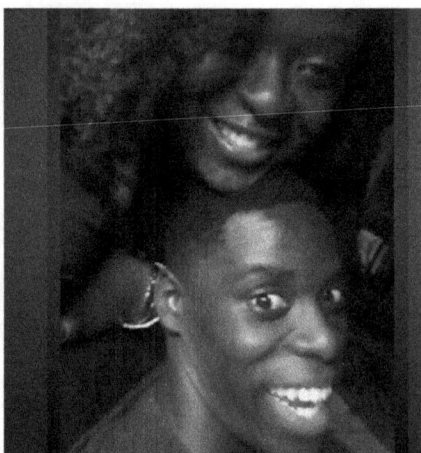

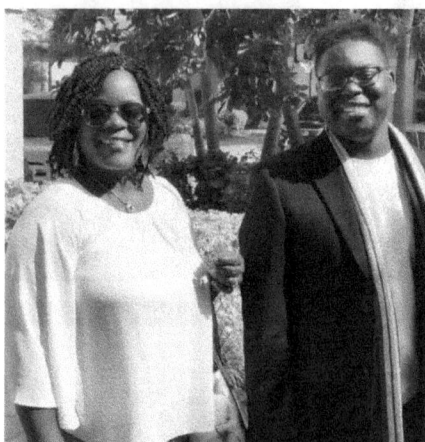

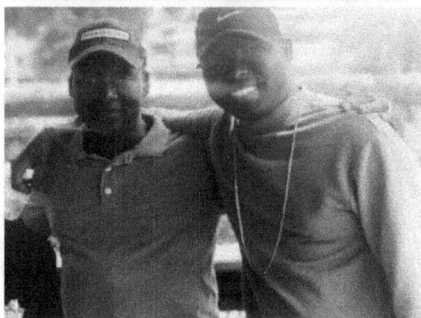

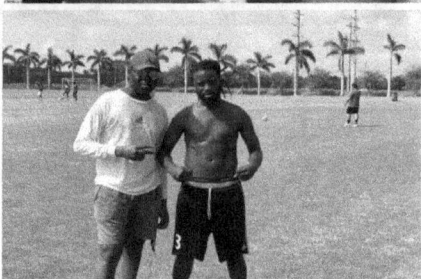

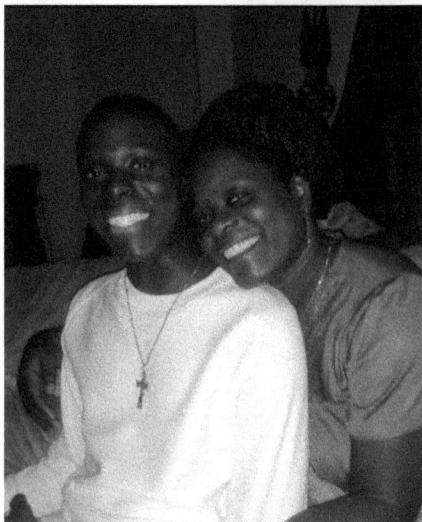

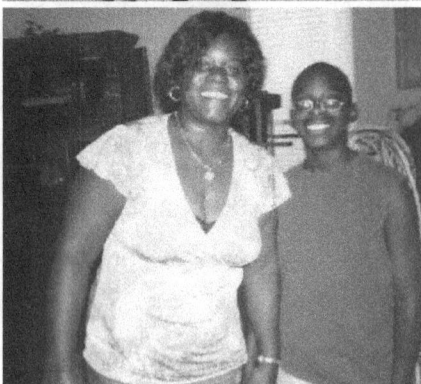

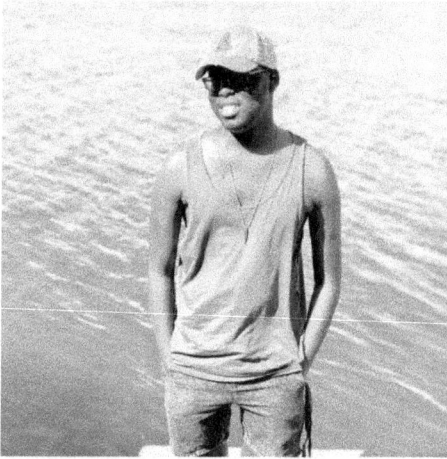
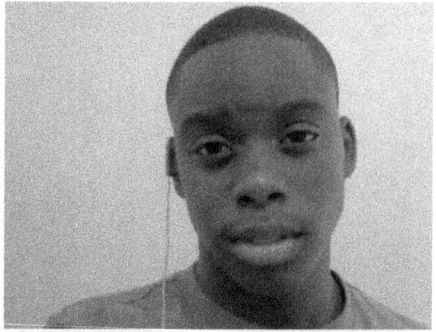
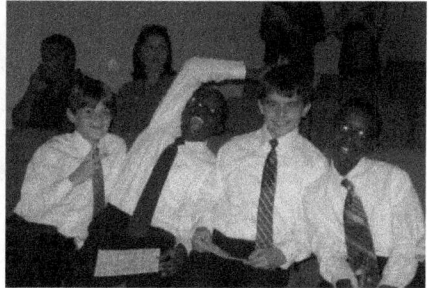
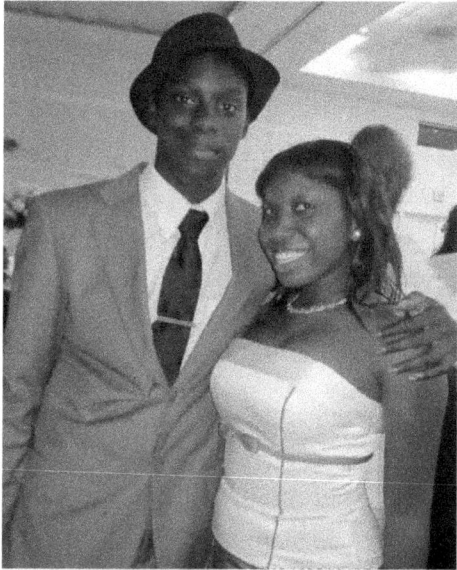
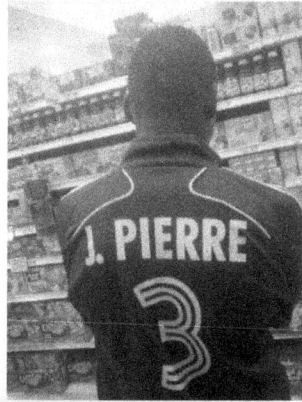
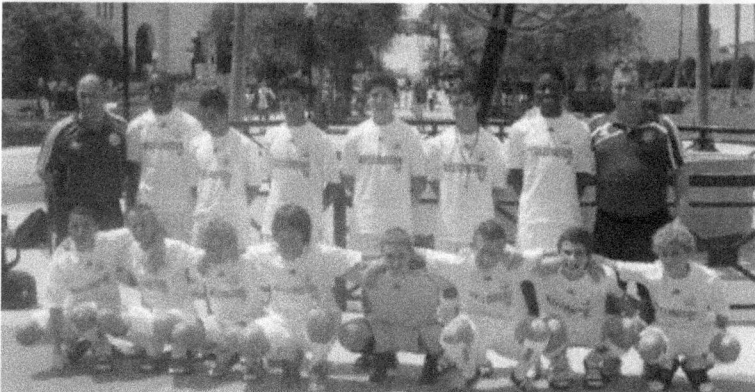

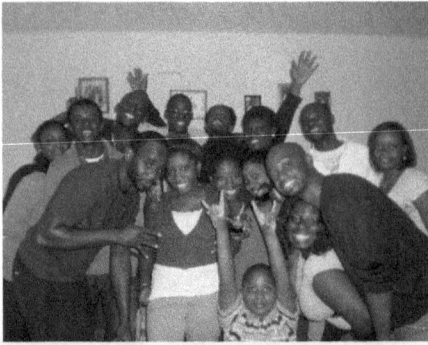
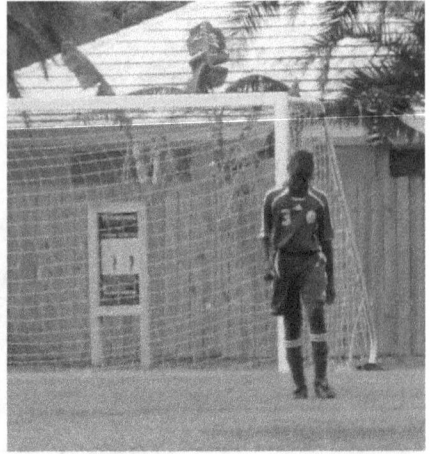
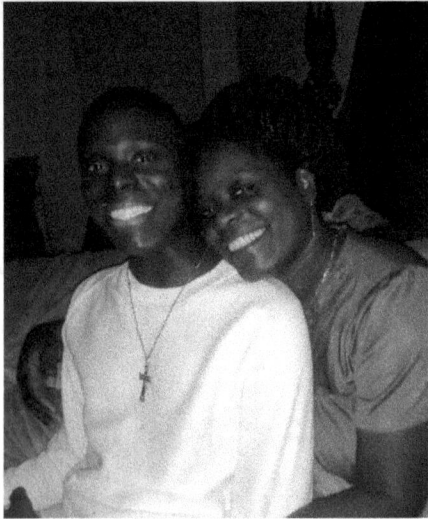
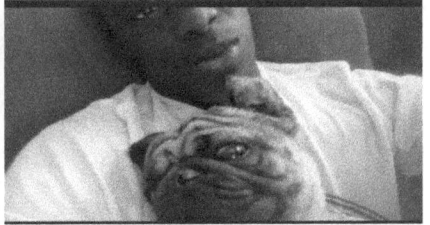
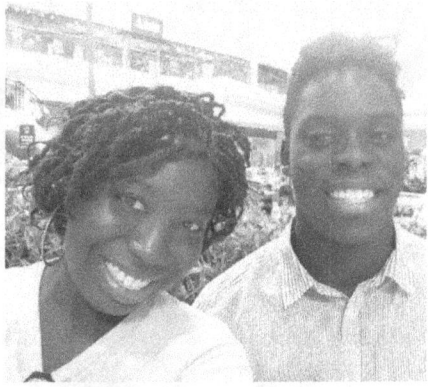
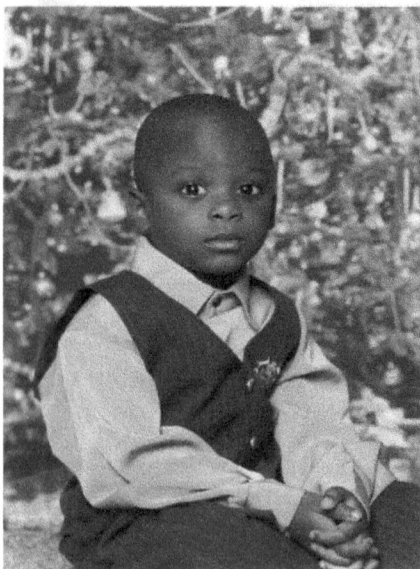
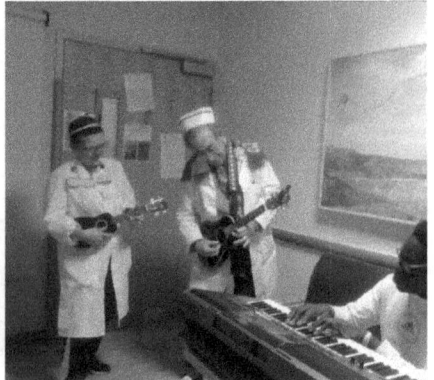

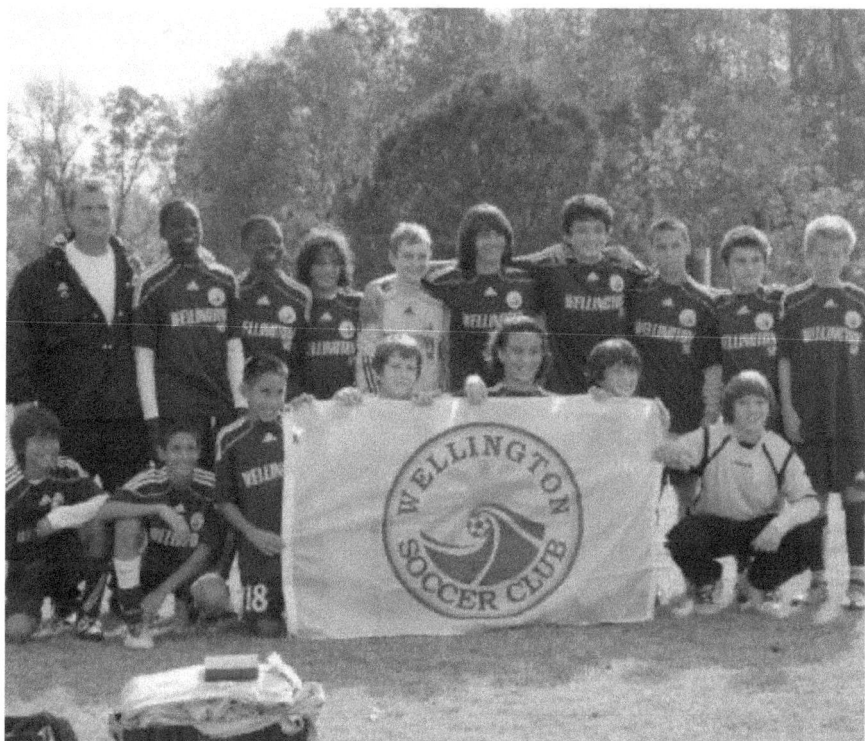

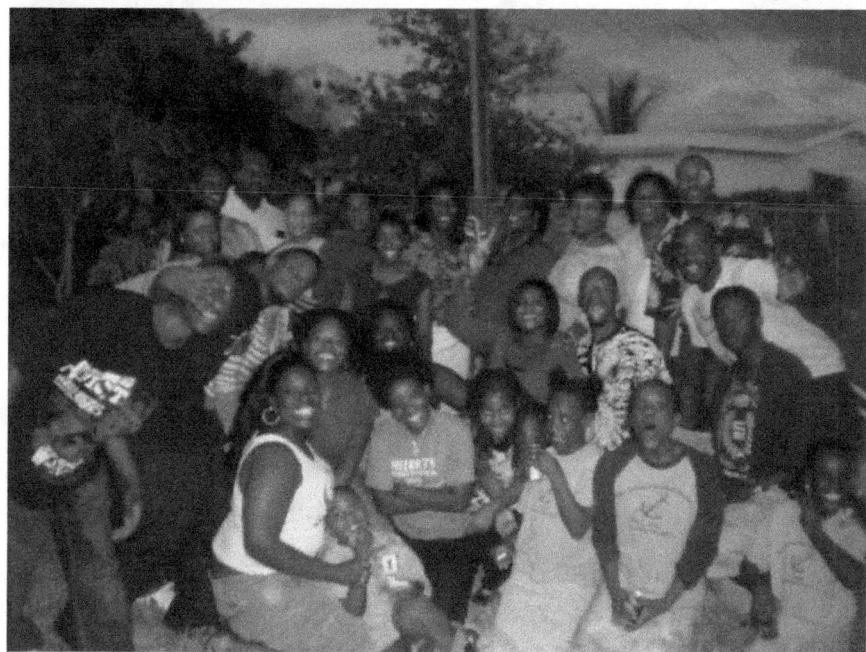

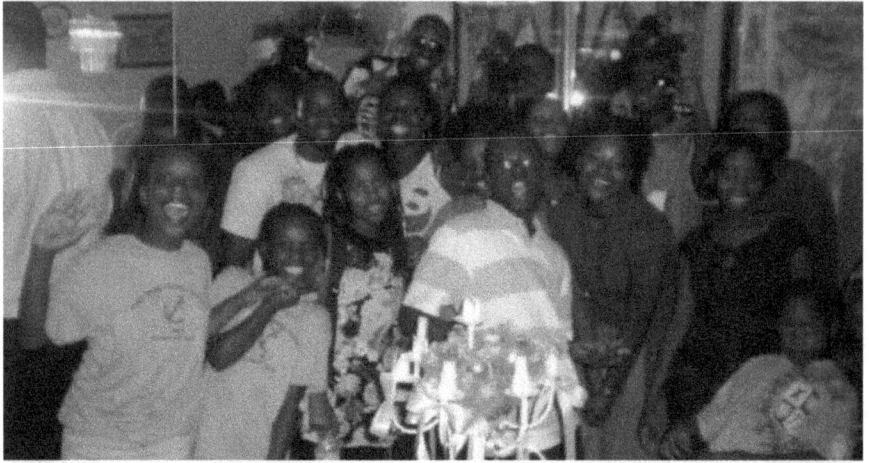
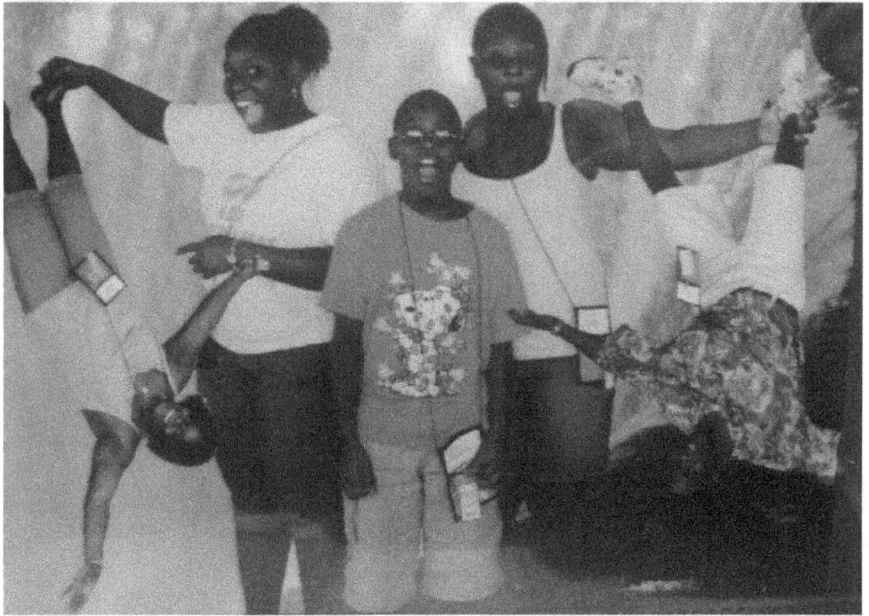

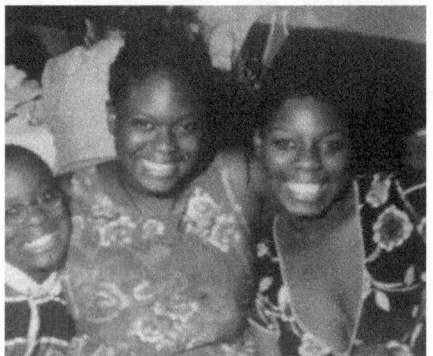

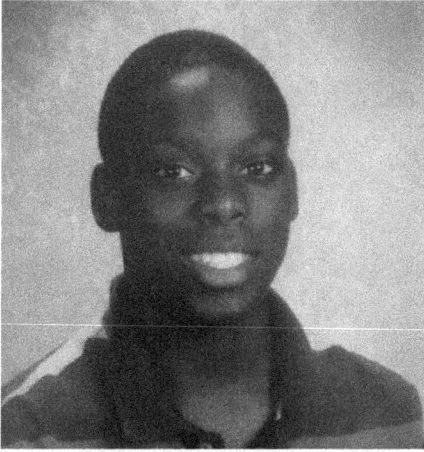
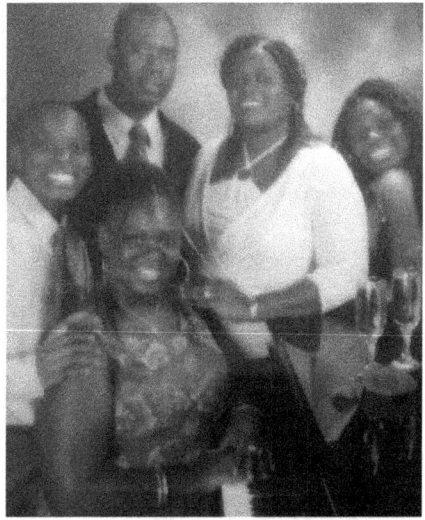
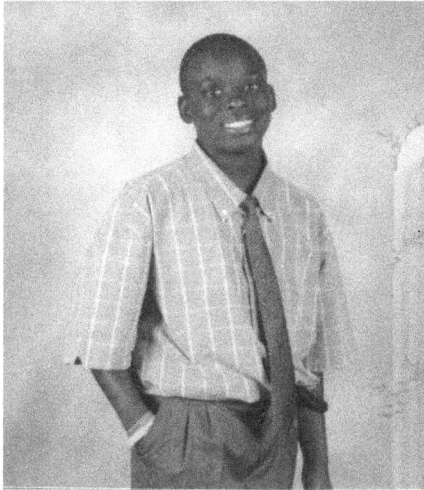
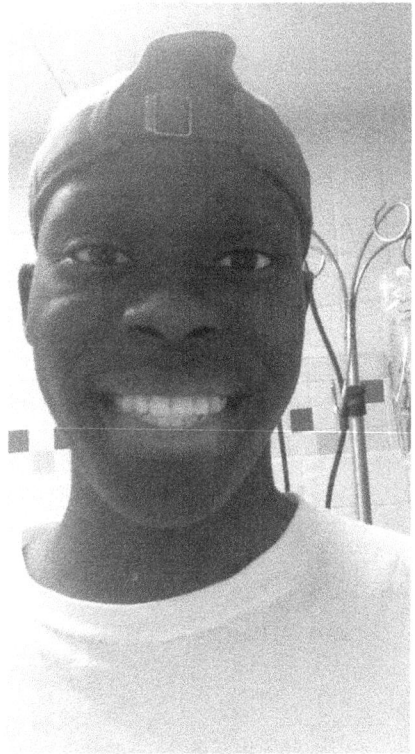
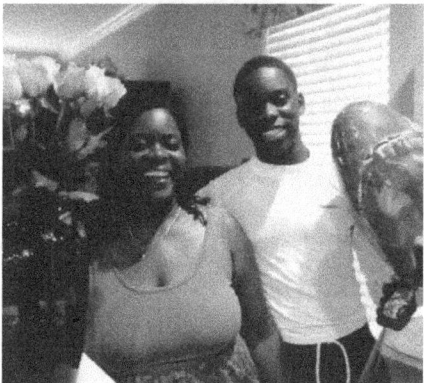

Jethro's Voice & Social Life

3 Birds 4 Life
Acceptance Video

Jethro's
YouTube Channel

SoundCloud Music

To listen to Jethro's
Shared Playlist on
SoundCloud

Jethro's IG

Jethro's Facebook

Jethro's Twitter

Jethro's Short Soccer Career Highlights

NCSA Sports

Sun Sentinel Article

SINCSPORTS

References and Citations

Popcorn Lung

PICC Line

Lumbar Puncture

Bone Marrow Transplant

Bone Marrow Biopsy

PET Scan

TV Quote

Complete References Appendix (Actual Web Links)

Jethro's Voice & Social Life

1. https://youtu.be/sPmdbBXHt5U
2. https://youtube.com/@jethropierre8301
3. https://soundcloud.com/jethropierre/popular-tracks
4. https://m.soundcloud.com/jethropierre
5. https://www.instagram.com/jethro_pierre
6. https://www.facebook.com/Jethro3rd
7. https://twitter.com/Jethro_Pierre

Jethro's Short Soccer Career Highlights

1. https://www.ncsasports.org/mens-soccer-recruiting/florida/west-palm-beach/palm-beach-city-high-school/jethro-pierre
2. https://www.sun-sentinel.com/sports/fl-xpm-2013-11-01-fl-palm-boys-soccer-preview-1103-20131101-story.html
3. https://soccer.sincsports.com/team/team

References and Citations

1. https://www.lung.org/lung-health-diseases/lung-disease-lookup/popcorn-lung/learn-about-popcorn-lung
2. https://www.mayoclinic.org/tests-procedures/picc-line/about/pac-20468748
3. https://www.mayoclinic.org/tests-procedures/lumbar-puncture/about/pac-20394631
4. https://www.mayoclinic.org/tests-procedures/bone-marrow-transplant/about/pac-20384854
5. https://www.mayoclinic.org/tests-procedures/bone-marrow-biopsy/about/pac-20393117
6. https://www.mayoclinic.org/tests-procedures/pet-scan/about/pac-20385078
7. https://tvquot.es/the-golden-girls/ebbtides-revenge/
8. https://www.palmswestfuneralhome.com/obituaries/Jethro-Pierre/

YOU WRITE, WE PUBLISH, TOGETHER WE CREATE

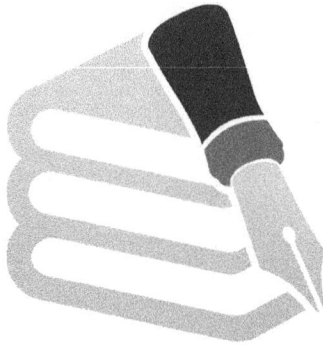

DIVINE WORKS PUBLISHING, LLC.

A co-publishing house for indie authors seeking a strategic bigger partner alliance for greater visibility and success in today's marketplace.

www.DivineWorksPublishing.com

561-990-BOOK (2665)

info@ DivineWorksPublishing.com